13 PRACTICAL WAYS TO HEAL FROM EMOTIONALLY IMMATURE PARENTS

ESSENTIAL TECHNIQUES TO REDUCE ANXIETY AND SET BOUNDARIES WITH NARCISSISTIC AND DYSFUNCTIONAL PARENTS

SILVIA M. DOUGH

TABLE OF CONTENTS

INTRODUCTION

THE INVISIBLE BURDEN WE CARRY

 "The greatest burden a child must bear is the unlived life of its parents." - Carl Jung

As the child of an emotionally immature parent, I know the weight of that burden all too well. The constant walking on eggshells, the persistent feeling of never being quite good enough, and the anxiety and self-doubt that permeate every aspect of your life—it's a heavy load to carry.

And I'm not alone. Studies indicate that growing up with emotionally immature parents can profoundly impact mental health into adulthood. This includes higher rates of depression and anxiety, difficulties in forming healthy relationships, and a chronic sense of emptiness or disconnection.

If you've picked up this book, chances are you're familiar with these struggles. Perhaps you've spent years feeling like you're always falling short, no matter how hard you try. Maybe you find yourself in relationships that leave you feeling drained and unfulfilled, or you're battling a voice in your head that constantly whispers, "You're not enough."

I want you to know that you are not alone, and more importantly, that healing is possible. Truly. I've witnessed it time and again in my work as a counselor, and I've experienced it myself. When we begin to

1

understand the roots of our pain, validate our own experiences and emotions, and learn healthier ways of relating to ourselves and others, remarkable changes can happen.

YOUR JOURNEY TO WHOLENESS

By picking up this book, you've already taken a powerful first step on the path to healing. Acknowledging the impact of emotional immaturity and seeking guidance is a profound act of courage and self-love. It's a declaration that you're ready to break free from old patterns and step into the joyful, authentic life you deserve.

In these pages, I'll guide you through the 13 transformative strategies that I've found most effective in my work with adult children of emotionally immature parents. These tools have helped my clients—and myself—move from merely surviving to truly thriving. You'll learn how to:

- Set healthy boundaries and communicate your needs with confidence
- Validate your own emotions and experiences
- Reframe the negative beliefs and self-talk that hold you back
- Cultivate self-compassion and learn to nurture your inner child
- Build meaningful, reciprocal relationships as an adult
- Process and release old pain, anger, and grief
- Find forgiveness and inner peace (regardless of whether your parents change)
- Embrace your authentic self and live with vulnerability and courage

I know the thought of diving into this work can feel daunting. Believe me, I've been there. The journey of healing isn't always easy, and there will likely be difficult emotions and challenges that arise. But I promise you this: it's so worth it. And you don't have to walk this path alone.

A PERSONAL AND PROFESSIONAL JOURNEY

So, who am I, and why am I so passionate about this work? As a counselor and the daughter of an emotionally immature mother, I know firsthand the challenges and triumphs of this healing journey.

My own battle with emotional immaturity began in childhood. Growing up with an emotionally volatile mother, I grappled with intense anxiety, constant self-doubt, and a crippling fear of abandonment. For years, I found myself in one-sided friendships and romantic relationships, desperately trying to earn love and prove my worth.

It wasn't until my late twenties, when I started therapy, that things began to shift. As I learned about concepts like boundaries, self-compassion, and reparenting, I started to view my story in a new light. I realized that my struggles weren't a reflection of my worth but were instead due to the emotional deficits I had grown up with. Most importantly, I discovered that I had the power to break free from those old patterns and start a new chapter.

Healing wasn't a linear process. There were setbacks, relapses into people-pleasing, and moments of feeling utterly lost. However, little by little, I began to find my footing. I learned to tune into my own needs and emotions, to set boundaries with love and firmness, and to extend myself the grace and understanding I had always craved from others. As I did, my world began to change in ways I had never imagined.

Fast forward more than a decade, and I've had the privilege of witnessing countless individuals go through the same transformative process. I've seen people who felt broken beyond repair find wholeness, peace, and a deep sense of self-love. I've watched relationships transform, careers flourish, and long-held dreams become reality. And it all starts with the same courageous first step that you've taken today.

Now, with over a decade of experience helping adult children of emotionally immature parents navigate their own healing journeys, I've distilled the most effective strategies and techniques into this comprehensive guide.

THE PATH FORWARD

So, what does the road ahead look like? In the coming chapters, we'll delve into the 13 fundamental practices for healing from emotional immaturity. You'll gain a clear understanding of what emotional immaturity truly is—and what it is not. You'll learn how it impacts us as both children and adults, and why it's crucial to break free from its grip.

We will explore essential skills such as self-validation, boundary setting, and effective communication. You'll develop a toolkit for navigating even the most challenging family dynamics with groundedness and grace. Through exercises, reflections, and real-world examples, you'll begin to transform your self-talk, release old resentments, and connect with your most authentic self.

By the end of our journey, my hope is that you will not only possess a roadmap for healing but also an unshakable sense of your own inherent worthiness. You'll be able to look in the mirror and see the strong, capable, and deeply lovable person you've always been. Each new day will greet you with profound hope, excitement, and self-compassion.

Healing is your birthright, dear reader. No matter your age or how deeply entrenched your patterns may seem, transformation is always possible. It can start right here, right now, within the pages of this book and the vastness of your own wise, resilient heart.

So take a deep breath, and turn the page. Your next chapter awaits.

CHAPTER 1

RECOGNIZING AND UNDERSTANDING THE EMOTIONALLY IMMATURE PARENT

 "The greatest discovery of my generation is that human beings can alter their lives by altering their attitudes of mind." - William James

D o you ever feel like you're walking on emotional eggshells around your parents? You're not alone. Understanding the behavior of emotionally immature parents is the first step toward reclaiming your emotional freedom. With both personal and professional experience in this area, I'm here to guide you on this journey of discovery and healing.

Like many of you, I grew up with an emotionally immature parent. My mother, despite her best intentions, was a whirlwind of unpredictable emotions. One moment, she'd be laughing and joking; the next, she'd be in tears over something as trivial as a broken plate. It was exhausting, confusing, and at times, terrifying.

For years, I believed this volatility was normal. After all, aren't all parents a bit unpredictable? It wasn't until I was well into adulthood, working as a human resources professional and exploring psychology as a personal interest, that I realized there was a name for what I had experienced: emotional immaturity. This revelation was both a relief and a challenge, propelling me onto a path of understanding and healing that I now share with others.

In this chapter, we'll examine what emotional immaturity in parents looks like, delve into its root causes, and explore how it impacts us as adult children. By picking up this book, you've already taken the first crucial step towards healing. Understanding is the key to freedom, and that's exactly what we're going to focus on together.

SIGNS AND SYMPTOMS OF EMOTIONAL IMMATURITY IN PARENTS

Let's start by identifying the signs of emotional immaturity in parents. It's like learning to spot storm clouds on the horizon – once you know what to look for, you'll be better prepared to navigate the emotional weather.

The Emotional Rollercoaster

First on our list is what I call the "emotional rollercoaster." Remember how I mentioned my mother could shift from laughter to tears in the blink of an eye? That's a classic sign of emotional immaturity. These parents exhibit moods that fluctuate rapidly and intensely, often without any apparent reason. One minute they're your best friend, the next they're giving you the silent treatment because you forgot to buy their favorite brand of cereal.

This inconsistency can be incredibly destabilizing for children. Imagine trying to build a house on shifting sands—that's what it feels like to grow up with a parent whose emotions are constantly in flux. It creates an environment of uncertainty and anxiety, where children are left unsure of what to expect or how to behave to maintain peace.

The "It's All About Me" Show

Next, we have what I like to call the "It's All About Me" show, starring your parents. Emotionally immature parents often have an uncanny ability to make everything about themselves. Did you get a promotion at work? They might claim it's because they pushed you so hard. Did you fail an exam? They might express how devastated they are, framing it as a reflection on their parenting.

This self-centeredness stems from an inability to separate their own identities and emotions from those of their children. It's as if they're the star of a show, and you're merely a supporting character. This dynamic can leave children feeling unseen, unheard, and invalidated.

The Guilt-Tripper Extraordinaire

Then there's the guilt-tripper extraordinaire. This is a particularly challenging aspect of emotional immaturity that many of us have struggled with. These parents are experts at making you feel guilty for, well, just about anything. "After all I've done for you..." becomes their battle cry. They wield guilt like a weapon, using it to manipulate you into doing what they want.

This behavior often stems from their own insecurities and fears of abandonment. However, the impact on children can be severe, leading to a lifetime of feeling responsible for others' emotions and struggling to set healthy boundaries.

The Emotional Avoider

Let's not forget the emotional avoiders. These parents flee from emotions as if chased by a pack of wild dogs. Any hint of conflict or deep conversation triggers a quick escape—vanishing faster than you can say "Let's talk about our feelings."

This avoidance manifests in various ways. Some parents might physically leave the room when emotions intensify. Others might switch the topic, turn on the TV, or even gaslight their children by denying there's anything worth discussing. This behavior teaches children that emotions are either frightening or insignificant, which can lead to difficulties in expressing and managing emotions later in life.

Immature Parents, Traumatized Kids: Impact on Children

You might be wondering, "Silvia, this all sounds familiar, but how does it affect the children?" I'm glad you asked. Growing up with emotionally immature parents is like trying to build a sandcastle during high tide—it's unstable, unpredictable, and no matter how hard you try, it keeps falling apart.

Children of emotionally immature parents often struggle with self-esteem issues. When your emotional needs are constantly overlooked or dismissed, it's easy to start believing that you're not worthy of love or attention. I remember feeling like an invisible girl, desperately trying to be seen and heard by my mother. This feeling of invisibility can persist into adulthood, affecting everything from personal relationships to professional aspirations.

Anxiety is another common side effect. When you're always walking on eggshells, never knowing what might trigger an emotional outburst, it's natural to develop a sense of hypervigilance. You become an emotional weather forecaster, always on the lookout for signs of an impending storm. This constant state of alert can be exhausting, leading to chronic anxiety and stress-related health issues.

And then there's the confusion. When a parent's behavior is inconsistent, it leaves a child feeling lost and unsure. It's like playing a game where the rules keep changing—frustrating and ultimately demoralizing. This confusion can manifest in adulthood as difficulty in decision-making or a constant second-guessing of one's own judgments and feelings.

Case Study: Sarah's Story

To illustrate these impacts, let me share a case study from my professional experience. I once worked with a young woman, whom we'll call Sarah. Sarah's mother was a classic example of emotional immaturity. One day, she'd shower Sarah with affection; the next, she'd give her the cold shoulder for no apparent reason.

Sarah grew up feeling constantly off-balance, never sure if she was loved. As an adult, she struggled with relationships, always waiting for the other shoe to drop, always anticipating abandonment. Her mother's inconsistency had ingrained in her the belief that love was unreliable and that she couldn't trust her own feelings or those of others.

Through our work together, Sarah began to recognize these patterns and understand their origins. This awareness was the first step on her journey toward healthier relationships and a stronger sense of self.

UNDERSTANDING THE ROOT CAUSES

Now that we've identified the signs of emotional immaturity, let's delve into the reasons behind it. Why do some parents end up emotionally stunted? It's like peeling back the layers of an onion—it might be uncomfortable, but it's essential to reach the core of the issue.

Childhood Experiences

First and foremost, let's consider childhood experiences. You know the saying, "Hurt people hurt people"? It often holds true for emotionally immature parents. Many grew up in households where their own emotional needs went unmet. It's as if they were given an emotional toolbox, but half the tools were missing.

Take my own mother, for example. As I grew older and began to unravel the mystery of her behavior, I learned about her own childhood. Her father passed away when she was young, and her mother, overwhelmed with grief and the responsibilities of single parenthood, became emotionally distant. My mother never learned how to properly process and express her emotions. It was like she was trying to speak a language she'd never been taught.

This intergenerational transmission of emotional immaturity is a common pattern. Without intervention or a conscious effort to change, people often parent in the way they were parented, perpetuating the cycle.

Societal and Cultural Factors

But it's not just about individual experiences. Sometimes, entire generations are shaped by historical events or societal norms. Consider this —if you grew up during a time of war, economic depression, or in a culture that valued stoicism over emotional expression, your opportunities to develop emotional maturity might have been severely limited.

It's like trying to grow a garden during a drought—not impossible, but certainly challenging.

For instance, many individuals who experienced the Great Depression developed a scarcity mindset that impacted their emotional availability to their children. Similarly, cultural norms that discourage emotional expression, particularly among men, can foster emotional immaturity that is passed down through generations.

Attachment Theory

There's a fascinating concept in psychology known as attachment theory that sheds light on the development of emotional maturity. Don't worry, I'll explain it in simple terms.

Attachment theory posits that the bond we form with our primary caregivers in infancy lays the foundation for our future relationships and emotional growth. If a child has a secure attachment—meaning their caregiver consistently responds to their needs—they are more likely to grow into emotionally mature adults.

However, if the attachment is insecure—perhaps because the caregiver is inconsistent, neglectful, or even abusive—it can result in emotional immaturity later in life. It's akin to building a house on a shaky foundation; it might look stable on the surface, but it's susceptible to cracks and instability.

Research has underscored the long-term impacts of these early attachment patterns. For instance, a study published in the *Journal of Personality and Social Psychology* demonstrated that attachment styles established in childhood persist into adulthood and significantly affect romantic relationships (Hazan & Shaver, 1987).

Cultural Influences

Cultural factors also play a significant role in emotional development. In some cultures, openly expressing emotions is seen as a sign of weakness. In others, certain emotions—like anger in women or sadness in men—are considered taboo. It's akin to playing a game of emotional Tetris where some pieces are off-limits.

I once worked with a client whose father was raised in a culture that strongly valued stoicism in men. Displaying any emotion other than anger was perceived as weak. Consequently, my client's father had a very limited emotional range—he was either stoic or angry, with no middle ground. It was like living with an emotional light switch that only had two settings: off or full blast.

Understanding these cultural influences can help us approach our parents' emotional immaturity with more empathy and insight. While it doesn't excuse their behavior, it can provide a clearer explanation.

OLD WOUNDS, FRESH SCARS: IMPACT ON ADULT CHILDREN

Now, let's talk about how all of this affects us as adults. Brace yourselves, because this might feel like looking into a mirror – sometimes uncomfortable, but ultimately revealing and empowering.

Emotional Vocabulary and Expression

Growing up with emotionally immature parents is like trying to learn a language from someone who only knows a few words. As a result, you end up with a limited emotional vocabulary, often struggling to identify and express your own feelings. It's like being an emotional tourist in your own life, always feeling a bit lost and out of place.

I recall a client of mine—let's call him Tom. Tom's parents were classic emotional avoiders. Any display of emotion in their household was met with awkward silence or a swift change of subject. As an adult, Tom found himself grappling with anxiety and depression, yet he was unable to articulate what he was feeling. It was as if he was experiencing life in black and white, while everyone else saw it in color.

This difficulty in recognizing and expressing emotions, known as alexithymia, has been linked to growing up in environments where emotions are neither validated nor discussed (Taylor et al., 1997).

Relationship Patterns

But it's not just about recognizing emotions. Growing up in an emotionally immature environment can also foster challenging behavioral patterns and relational difficulties. It's as if we're given a faulty blueprint for relationships, and we keep constructing the same unstable structure repeatedly.

One common pattern is the fear of abandonment. When you've been raised by parents whose love felt conditional or inconsistent, you might find yourself perpetually anxious in relationships. It's like playing a game of emotional Jenga, always on edge, bracing for everything to collapse.

On the flip side, some adult children of emotionally immature parents veer towards the other extreme. They become fiercely independent, shunning deep connections. It's a classic case of "I'll leave you before you can leave me." It's like erecting a fortress around your heart—safe, but profoundly lonely.

Then there's the tendency to people-please. If you've grown accustomed to managing your parents' emotions, you might find yourself doing the same in all your relationships. It's like being a human mood ring, constantly adjusting to suit others, never quite sure of your own true color.

The Cycle of Emotional Immaturity

But here's where it gets really interesting—and a bit ironic. Many adult children of emotionally immature parents end up, wait for it, emotionally immature themselves. I know, plot twist, right? It's like we're actors who've been handed a bad script—we keep reciting the same lines, even though we know they don't sound quite right.

This manifestation of emotional immaturity in adulthood can take many forms. Maybe you find yourself overreacting to minor setbacks. Or perhaps you struggle with taking responsibility for your actions, always looking to blame someone else. It could even show up as difficulty in setting and respecting boundaries—after all, how can you set boundaries when you've never seen them modeled?

I'll never forget the day I realized I was exhibiting some of these behaviors myself. There I was, a professional in human resources, priding myself on my emotional intelligence, when I caught myself in a full-blown tantrum over a minor disagreement with my partner. It was like looking in a mirror and seeing my mother's face staring back at me. Talk about a wake-up call!

The Silver Lining

But here's the really good news: Awareness is the first step towards change. Once we recognize these patterns, we have the power to alter them. It's like being given a new pair of glasses—suddenly, everything becomes clear, and we have the choice to walk a different path.

Moreover, many adult children of emotionally immature parents develop remarkable strengths. They are often highly empathetic, intuitive, and resilient. It's as if they've been through an emotional boot camp—it was tough, but it made them stronger. Research has indicated that some individuals who face adversity in childhood experience what psychologists call "posttraumatic growth," which leads to increased personal strength and a deeper appreciation for life (Tedeschi & Calhoun, 2004).

As we wrap up this chapter, I want you to remember this: your past does not define your future. Yes, growing up with emotionally immature parents leaves its mark, but you have the power to heal, to grow, and to break the cycle. It's like you've been given a plot of land with poor soil—it might take more work to cultivate a garden, but the beauty of the blooms will be incredibly rewarding when they finally appear.

In Chapter 2, we're going to start the healing process by learning to accept our own emotions and feelings. After all, you can't pour from an empty cup, and emotional healing begins with self-acceptance. So, take a deep breath, give yourself a pat on the back for making it this far, and get ready to embark on the next step of our journey. Trust me, it's going to be transformative!

CHAPTER 1 TAKEAWAYS:

• Emotional immaturity in parents is characterized by unpredictable mood swings, self-centeredness, guilt-tripping, and emotional avoidance.

• Signs of emotionally immature parents include:

- Rapid and intense mood fluctuations

- Making everything about themselves

- Using guilt as a manipulation tactic

- Avoiding emotional discussions or confrontations

• Growing up with emotionally immature parents can lead to:

- Low self-esteem and feelings of invisibility

- Chronic anxiety and hypervigilance

- Confusion about one's own emotions and needs

• Root causes of parental emotional immaturity often include:

- Their own unmet childhood emotional needs

- Generational patterns of emotional neglect

- Societal and cultural factors that discourage emotional expression

- Insecure attachment styles formed in early childhood

• The impact on adult children can manifest as:

- Difficulty identifying and expressing emotions (alexithymia)

- Challenging relationship patterns, including fear of abandonment or extreme independence

- People-pleasing tendencies

- Potential to repeat patterns of emotional immaturity

• Understanding these patterns is the first step towards breaking the cycle of emotional immaturity.

• Many adult children of emotionally immature parents develop strengths such as empathy, intuition, and resilience.

• Awareness of these patterns opens the door to personal growth and healing.

• Remember: Your past does not define your future. You have the power to heal and create healthier emotional patterns.

CHAPTER 2

THE BITTER PILL: ACCEPTING YOUR EMOTIONS AND FEELINGS

"The emotion that can break your heart is sometimes the very one that heals it." - Nicholas Sparks

Emotions are the language of the soul, yet accepting them can be one of the toughest challenges we face, especially when our upbringing taught us otherwise. Embrace your emotions; they hold the key to your healing.

Growing up with emotionally immature parents, I learned to bottle up my feelings. I became a master at emotional suppression, believing it was essential for survival in a household where my emotions were often dismissed or ridiculed. However, this strategy backfired spectacularly.

I remember the day it all came crashing down. While at work, submerged in a sea of spreadsheets, a colleague made a harmless joke about my meticulousness. Suddenly, I was hit by a tidal wave of emotions—anger, shame, sadness—all threatening to overwhelm me. My hands shook, my vision blurred, and before I knew it, I found myself sobbing in a bathroom stall, bewildered by what was happening.

That breakdown marked the beginning of my breakthrough. It forced me to confront the emotions I had been suppressing for years and set me on a path toward emotional healing. This chapter aims to share the transformative power of accepting your emotions and feelings.

EMOTIONAL AWARENESS: WHY IT MATTERS

Imagine trying to navigate a complex maze blindfolded. That's what life can feel like without emotional awareness. You bump into walls, make wrong turns, and end up frustrated and lost. But once the blindfold is removed, the path ahead becomes clear.

Emotional awareness is your inner compass, guiding you through life's challenges. It allows you to recognize and understand your emotions as they occur. Truly, it's a game-changer.

Research supports this. A study published in the Journal of Personality and Social Psychology found that individuals with higher emotional awareness reported lower levels of stress and better overall well-being (Barrett et al., 2001). It's akin to possessing a superpower—the ability to understand and navigate your emotional landscape with precision.

However, many of us who grew up with emotionally immature parents never developed this crucial awareness. We learned to ignore our feelings, suppress them, or wear masks of perpetual okayness. While these strategies might have helped us cope then, they now serve as barriers to our growth.

How Emotional Suppression Leads to Stress and Anxiety

Think of emotional suppression as a pressure cooker. You keep adding ingredients (emotions) and turning up the heat (stress), but never release the valve. What happens? Eventually, it explodes, leaving a mess everywhere.

I lived this reality for years. I prided myself on my ability to "keep it together" in any situation. But inside, I was a roiling mass of unexpressed emotions. The result? Chronic anxiety, tension headaches, and a constant feeling of being on edge.

A study in the Journal of Abnormal Psychology demonstrated that chronic emotional suppression is linked to higher rates of anxiety and depression (Gross & Levenson, 1997). It's not just detrimental to your mental health—it also takes a toll on your physical well-being.

So, how do we build this emotional awareness? It starts with learning to identify and label our emotions. This might sound simple, but for many of us, it's akin to learning a new language.

Here's an exercise I found incredibly helpful:

The Emotion Check-In; Throughout the day, pause and ask yourself, "What am I feeling right now?" Don't judge the emotion, just observe it. Is it anger? Sadness? Joy? Fear? The more you practice this, the more fluent you'll become in your emotional language.

Another technique is keeping an **Emotion Journal** and at the end of each day, jot down the emotions you experienced. Over time, you'll start to see patterns and triggers, giving you valuable insights into your emotional landscape.

Mindfulness Practices to Enhance Emotional Awareness

Mindfulness isn't just a buzzword; it's a powerful tool for enhancing emotional awareness. It involves being present in the moment, observing your thoughts and feelings without judgment.

I was initially skeptical. Sit still and focus on my breath? It seemed unlikely. However, as I continued to practice, I noticed a shift. I became more attuned to the subtle emotions I had previously ignored. It was like turning up the volume on my inner world.

Try this simple mindfulness exercise: Set a timer for five minutes. Close your eyes and focus on your breath. When thoughts or emotions arise (and they will), acknowledge them without judgment and gently return your focus to your breathing. It's not about clearing your mind; it's about observing what's there.

EMBRACING VULNERABILITY: THE COURAGE TO FEEL

In a world that often equates vulnerability with weakness, embracing our emotions can feel downright scary. But here's the truth bomb: vulnerability is not weakness. It's courage in its purest form.

How Vulnerability Fosters Emotional Growth

Brené Brown, a researcher who's spent years studying vulnerability, puts it beautifully: **"Vulnerability is the birthplace of innovation, creativity and change."** When we allow ourselves to be vulnerable, to really feel our emotions, we open ourselves up to profound growth and connection.

I remember the first time I allowed myself to be truly vulnerable. I was having coffee with a close friend and, instead of giving my usual "I'm fine" when she asked how I was, I told her the truth. I shared my fears, insecurities, and struggles with my parents. Instead of judgment, I received empathy and support. That moment of vulnerability deepened our friendship and made me feel less alone in my struggles.

But let's be real—vulnerability can feel terrifying, especially if you've grown up in an environment where your emotions were dismissed or used against you. The shame associated with feelings can be a heavy burden.

I carried that shame for years, believing that my emotions made me weak, that they were something to be hidden away. However, as I've learned to accept and express my feelings, I've discovered that they are not a weakness—they are a strength.

Here's a powerful exercise for overcoming shame: Write a letter to your emotions. Thank them for what they're trying to tell you. Apologize for ignoring or suppressing them. This exercise might feel silly at first, but it can be incredibly healing.

DEVELOPING A HEALTHY EMOTIONAL RESPONSE

Now that we've talked about awareness and vulnerability, let's go into developing a healthy emotional response. This is where the rubber meets the road in our journey of healing.

When you're in the grip of a strong feeling, it can feel like you're being swept away by a tidal wave. But there are ways to ride that wave instead of being overwhelmed by it.

One technique I've found incredibly helpful is the RAIN method, developed by psychologist Tara Brach:

- Recognize what's happening
- Allow the experience to be there, just as it is
- Investigate with interest and care
- Nurture with self-compassion

Let me give you an example. A few months ago, I received some harsh criticism at work. My immediate reaction was a mix of anger and shame. Instead of lashing out or shutting down, I tried the RAIN method:

1. I recognized that I was feeling hurt and defensive.

2. I allowed those feelings to be there, without trying to push them away.

3. Reaching out and finding out where I could have improved

4. I acknowledged the importance of being kind to myself and accepted that it's okay to feel hurt. I reminded myself that criticism is an opportunity for growth, and I offered myself compassion and encouragement as I worked on improving.

By following these steps, we can start to break free from the grip of shame and embrace our authentic selves. It's not an easy process, but it's incredibly liberating. Remember, your feelings are valid, and you have nothing to be ashamed of.

Strategies for Building Emotional Resilience

Now that we've talked about vulnerability and shame, let's talk about building emotional resilience. Think of emotional resilience as your inner bouncy castle – no matter how hard life knocks you down, you've got the ability to bounce back up.

Here are some strategies I've found helpful in building emotional resilience:

1. **Practice Self-Compassion:** Treat yourself with the same kindness you'd offer a good friend. When you're struggling, ask yourself, "What would I say to a friend in this situation?" Then say those words to yourself.

2. **Develop a Growth Mindset**: Instead of seeing challenges as failures, view them as opportunities for learning and growth. Ask yourself, "What can I learn from this experience?"

3. **Build a Support Network**: Surround yourself with people who uplift and encourage you. Remember, you don't have to go through this journey alone.

4. **Cultivate Mindfulness:** Regular mindfulness practice can help you stay grounded in the present moment, rather than getting caught up in worries about the future or regrets about the past.

5. **Practice Gratitude:** Take time each day to notice and appreciate the good things in your life, no matter how small they might seem.

Coping Mechanisms for Managing Intense Emotions

When intense emotions hit, it can feel like you're caught in a tornado. But with the right coping mechanisms, you can weather the storm. Here are some techniques I've found helpful:

1. **The 5-4-3-2-1 Grounding Technique:** When you're feeling over-whelmed, focus on:

- 5 things you can see

- 4 things you can touch

- 3 things you can hear

- 2 things you can smell

- 1 thing you can taste

This technique helps bring you back to the present moment and out of the emotional whirlwind.

2. **Box Breathing:** Imagine tracing a square in your mind. As you trace each side, count to four. Inhale for 4, hold for 4, exhale for 4, hold for 4. Repeat as needed.

3. **Emotional Surfing**: Instead of trying to push away intense emotions, imagine yourself surfing on the waves of your feelings. Observe them rise and fall without getting swept away.

4. **The STOP Technique:**

- Stop what you're doing

- Take a breath

- Observe your thoughts and feelings

- Proceed mindfully

Remember, the goal isn't to eliminate intense emotions – they're a natural part of life. The goal is to learn how to ride the waves without drowning.

Techniques for Self-Soothing and Self-Care

Self-soothing is like having a first-aid kit for your emotions. It's about nurturing yourself through difficult times. Here are some self-soothing techniques you can try:

1. **Create a Comfort Box:** Fill a box with items that engage your senses and bring you comfort. This could include a soft blanket, a scented candle, a favorite book, or photos of happy memories.

2. **Practice Progressive Muscle Relaxation**: Starting from your toes and working up to your head, tense each muscle group for 5 seconds, then release. Notice the difference between tension and relaxation.

3. **Use Positive Self-Talk:** Develop a list of comforting phrases you can say to yourself in times of distress. For example, "This feeling will pass," or "I am safe and capable."

4. **Engage in Creative Expression**: Whether it's drawing, writing, dancing, or singing, creative activities can be incredibly soothing and help process emotions.

Let me share a personal story with you. A few years ago, I was preparing for a big presentation at work. The night before, I felt an overwhelming wave of anxiety. Previously, I would have pushed those feelings aside, telling myself to "toughen up." But this time, I tried something different.

I acknowledged my anxiety, telling myself, "I'm feeling anxious, and that's okay." I used the box breathing technique to calm my nerves and then journaled about my fears, which helped me realize that my anxiety stemmed from a desire to do well—a completely normal feeling!

By accepting my emotions instead of fighting them, I was able to channel that energy into preparation. The presentation went better than I could have imagined, and I gained a newfound sense of confidence in my ability to handle stress.

Another example involves a client of mine, let's call her Liza. Liza grew up with a mother who often dismissed her feelings, telling her to "stop being so sensitive." As a result, Liza struggled with emotional numbness in her adult relationships.

Through our work together, Liza began practicing emotional awareness and acceptance. Initially, it was challenging—she often couldn't differentiate between sadness and anger, or anxiety and excitement.

However, with practice, Liza became more attuned to her emotional landscape. She started journaling daily, which helped her notice patterns in her feelings and behaviors. She also began practicing mindfulness meditation, which allowed her to stay present with her emotions without judgment.

The turning point for Liza came when she expressed her hurt and disappointment to her partner after a disagreement, instead of shutting down as she usually did. This vulnerable expression led to a deeper connection in her relationship and a sense of empowerment in her emotional life.

These examples illustrate that emotional acceptance is not about controlling or eliminating our feelings. It's about acknowledging them, understanding them, and allowing them to guide us rather than control us.

As we wrap up this chapter, remember that accepting your emotions is a journey, not a destination. There will be days when it feels easier and days when it's a struggle. That's okay. What matters is that you're taking steps towards a more emotionally aware and authentic life.

In Chapter 3, we'll explore how to choose your battles wisely when dealing with emotionally immature parents. We'll discuss strategies for identifying which issues are worth addressing and how to conserve your emotional energy for the things that truly matter. Remember, every step you take in understanding and accepting your emotions is a step towards healing and growth. You've got this!

CHAPTER TAKEAWAYS:

- Emotional awareness is crucial for healing from parental emotional immaturity. It's like having a GPS for your inner world.
- Emotional suppression leads to increased stress and anxiety. It's like a pressure cooker that eventually explodes.
- Techniques for identifying and labeling emotions, such as the Emotion Check-In and Emotion Journal, can help build emotional awareness.
- Mindfulness practices enhance emotional awareness by helping us observe our thoughts and feelings without judgment.

- Embracing vulnerability fosters emotional growth. It's not weakness, but courage in its purest form.
- Overcoming shame associated with feelings is essential. Our emotions are not a weakness, but a strength.
- Building emotional resilience involves practicing self-compassion, cultivating a growth mindset, building a support network, and engaging in regular self-care.
- The RAIN method (Recognize, Allow, Investigate, Nurture) is a powerful tool for managing intense emotions.
- Self-soothing techniques and self-care practices are crucial for maintaining emotional health.
- Emotional acceptance doesn't make negative feelings disappear, but it changes our relationship with our emotions, allowing for more resilient responses to life's challenges.

CHAPTER 3
CHOOSING YOUR BATTLES

 "The art of war teaches us to rely not on the likelihood of the enemy not coming, but on our own readiness to receive him; not on the chance of his not attacking, but rather on the fact that we have made our position unassailable." - Sun Tzu

Every interaction is a battle, but not all battles are worth fighting. Learning to choose your battles wisely with emotionally immature parents can save you both energy and emotional turmoil.

I recall the days when I would get worked up over every little comment my mom made about my appearance or my career choices. It was exhausting, like trying to plug a dam with my bare hands while the water kept rushing in. But then I realized something crucial—I was wasting my energy on battles that weren't moving me forward. That realization was a game-changer. I started to strategize my interactions, which dramatically shifted the dynamics.

In this chapter, we will delve deep into the art of selective engagement. Think of it as your personal battle plan for minimizing conflict and stress when dealing with emotionally immature parents. We'll explore how to identify triggers, establish priorities in communication, and maintain that oh-so-important emotional detachment. By the end of this chapter, you'll be equipped with the tools to navigate these tricky waters with the finesse of a seasoned diplomat.

IDENTIFYING TRIGGERS AND PATTERNS

You're sitting at the dinner table, enjoying a peaceful meal, when suddenly your dad comments on your weight. Instantly, you feel your blood pressure rise and your jaw clench, and before you know it, you're in the middle of a full-blown argument. Sound familiar?

Recognizing these situations is like developing a sixth sense for emotional landmines. It involves becoming aware of the subtle cues that signal an impending storm. Maybe it's the way your mom purses her lips when she's about to critique your parenting style, or the particular tone your dad adopts when he's about to lecture you on your career choices.

For me, it was my mother's habitual preface of "I'm just saying..." I learned that whatever followed was almost guaranteed to push my buttons. Once I recognized this pattern, I could mentally prepare myself or even steer the conversation in a different direction before things escalated.

Now, let's talk about those pesky triggers. These are the hot-button issues that seem to ignite conflict faster than a match to gasoline. Based on my experience and research, here are some common triggers when dealing with emotionally immature parents:

1. Criticism of life choices (career, relationships, parenting)

2. Unsolicited advice

3. Comparisons to siblings or other family members

4. Guilt-tripping or emotional manipulation

5. Dismissal of feelings or experiences

6. Invasion of privacy or boundaries

Dr. Lindsay Gibson, in her book Adult Children of *Emotionally Immature Parents*, highlights that these triggers often stem from unresolved childhood issues. She explains, "Emotionally immature parents tend to repeat patterns of behavior that worked for them in the past, even if those patterns are no longer effective or appropriate" (Gibson, 2015).

Understanding these triggers is akin to having a map of the emotional battlefield. It allows you to anticipate potential conflicts and prepare yourself accordingly.

Now that we've identified the triggers, let's talk strategy. Preemptive conflict resolution is all about nipping potential arguments in the bud before they have a chance to bloom into full-blown confrontations. Here are some techniques I've found effective:

1. **The Redirect:** When you sense a triggering topic approaching, gently steer the conversation in a different direction. For example, if your mom starts critiquing your parenting, you might say, "Oh, that reminds me, I've been meaning to ask you about that recipe you used to make when we were kids."

2. **The Acknowledge and Move On:** Sometimes, a simple acknowledgment can defuse a situation. "I understand you're concerned about my career choices, Mom. I appreciate your input. Now, tell me about your garden - how are those tomatoes coming along?"

3. **The Time-Out**: If you feel tensions rising, it's okay to excuse yourself for a moment. A quick trip to the restroom or to get a glass of water can give you the breather you need to reset.

4. **The Empathy Approach**: Try to understand where your parents are coming from, even if you disagree. "I can see why you might be worried about my decision, Dad. It's because you care about my well-being, right?"

5. **The Boundary Setting:** Sometimes, you need to be direct. "I know you have strong opinions about this, Mom, but I've made my decision and I'm not open to discussing it further right now."

Remember, the goal here isn't to win an argument, but to prevent unnecessary conflict. As the old saying goes, an ounce of prevention is worth a pound of cure.

ESTABLISHING PRIORITIES IN COMMUNICATION

Now that we've covered identifying triggers and preemptive strategies, let's discuss prioritizing our battles. Not all issues are created equal, and learning to differentiate between minor annoyances and major concerns is crucial for maintaining your sanity.

Here's a hard truth I had to accept: you can't change your parents. I know—it's a tough pill to swallow. I spent years trying to make my mom understand my perspective, hoping that clear enough explanations might lead to an "aha" moment and transform her into the emotionally mature parent I'd always wanted.

However, expecting significant changes from emotionally immature parents is like expecting a cat to bark. It's simply not in their nature. Dr. Joshua Coleman, a psychologist specializing in adult child-parent relationships, notes in his book Rules of Estrangement that "Parents who struggle with emotional immaturity often have deeply ingrained patterns of behavior that are resistant to change" (Coleman, 2021).

What does this mean for us? It means we need to adjust our expectations. Instead of hoping for a complete personality overhaul, we should aim for small improvements in our interactions. Perhaps your dad won't suddenly become a great listener, but he might learn to hold his tongue more often if you consistently enforce your boundaries.

Remember, setting realistic expectations isn't about giving up hope. It's about focusing your energy where it can make a difference—on your own responses and behaviors.

Techniques for Prioritizing Issues Worth Addressing

Not every battle needs to be fought, and not every issue needs to be addressed. Learning to prioritize is like becoming the CEO of your own emotional well-being. Here's how you can decide what's worth your time and energy:

1. **The Impact Test**: Ask yourself, "How much does this issue impact my daily life and overall well-being?" If it's a minor annoyance that you can brush off, it might not be worth addressing.

2. **The Frequency Factor:** Is this a one-off incident or a recurring problem? Persistent issues that keep cropping up might need to be addressed.

3. **The Change Potential:** Consider whether addressing this issue has the potential to lead to positive change. Some battles aren't worth fighting if the outcome is likely to be the same regardless.

4. **The Emotional Cost:** Weigh the emotional toll of addressing the issue against the potential benefits. Sometimes, letting something go is less stressful than confronting it.

5. **The Boundary Check**: Does this issue involve a violation of your personal boundaries? These are often worth addressing to maintain your self-respect and emotional health.

How to Communicate Effectively Without Escalating Conflicts

Now that we've identified our priority issues, let's talk about how to address them without turning every conversation into World War III. Effective communication with emotionally immature parents is an art form, but with practice, you can become a master.

1. **Use "I" Statements**: Instead of saying "You always criticize me;" try "I feel hurt when my choices are criticized." This approach is less accusatory and more likely to be heard.

2. **Choose Your Timing Wisely:** Don't try to have important conversations when emotions are already running high. Pick a calm moment when both you and your parents are in a good headspace.

3. **Stay Calm and Composed**: Remember, you're the emotionally mature one here. Take deep breaths, speak slowly, and keep your tone even.

4. **Be Specific**: Instead of generalizing ("You never listen to me"), provide concrete examples ("When I was talking about my promotion yesterday, I felt like you were dismissing my accomplishments").

5. **Listen Actively:** Show that you're listening by paraphrasing what your parents say. This doesn't mean you agree, but it shows you're making an effort to understand.

6. **Set Clear Boundaries:** Be firm but kind when establishing limits. "I'm not comfortable discussing my weight. Let's talk about something else."

7. **Use the Sandwich Method**: When addressing a difficult topic, sandwich it between two positive statements. For example, "I appreciate your concern for my wellbeing. I need you to respect my career choices. I know it comes from a place of love."

Remember, effective communication is a two-way street. You might not always get the response you're hoping for, but by maintaining your composure and expressing yourself clearly, you're setting a positive example.

Maintaining Emotional Detachment

This doesn't mean becoming cold or uncaring. Think of it more as creating a healthy emotional buffer zone - like wearing a raincoat in a storm. You're still there, you still care, but you're not getting soaked by every emotional downpour.

Tools for Emotional Distancing During Challenging Interactions

1. **The Mental Bubble:** Imagine yourself surrounded by a protective bubble. Negative comments or behaviors bounce off this bubble instead of penetrating your emotional core.

2. **The Observer Technique:** Pretend you're a scientist observing an interesting specimen. This can help you maintain objectivity and reduce emotional reactivity.

3. **The Mantra Method**: Develop a personal mantra to repeat silently

during tense moments. Something like "This is their issue, not mine" or "I choose peace over conflict" can be grounding.

4. **The Breathing Anchor:** Focus on your breath during challenging interactions. Count your inhales and exhales to stay centered and calm.

5. **The Time Travel Trick**: Imagine yourself a week, a month, or a year from now. Will this interaction still matter? This perspective can help reduce immediate emotional intensity.

Setting Boundaries on Emotional Involvement

Setting boundaries isn't just about what you say or do - it's also about protecting your emotional energy. Here are some strategies to help you maintain a healthy level of emotional involvement:

1. **The Emotional Bank Account**: Imagine you have a limited amount of emotional currency to spend each day. Budget it wisely, saving some for self-care and personal relationships.

2. **The Role Definition**: Remind yourself that you're the child, not the parent. It's not your job to manage their emotions or solve their problems.

3. **The Empathy Limit**: While empathy is important, too much can be draining. It's okay to say, "I understand you're upset, but I don't have the capacity to discuss this right now."

4. **The Self-Check In:** Regularly ask yourself, "How am I feeling right now?" If you're becoming too emotionally invested, it might be time to step back.

5. **The Support System Utilization:** Lean on friends, partners, or therapists for emotional support instead of getting overly involved with your parents' issues.

Dr. Karyl McBride, author of "Will I Ever Be Good Enough? Healing the Daughters of Narcissistic Mothers," emphasizes the importance of emotional boundaries: "Setting emotional boundaries is about taking responsibility for your own feelings while letting others take responsibility for theirs" (McBride, 2008).

CASE STUDIES ILLUSTRATING EFFECTIVE CONFLICT RESOLUTION STRATEGIES

Let's bring all of this together with some real-life examples. These case studies are composites based on my experiences and those of my clients, with names and details changed to protect privacy.

Case Study 1: The Holiday Dilemma

Amy always dreaded the holidays because her mother, Linda, would guilt-trip her about not spending enough time with the family. This year, Amy decided to apply the techniques we've discussed.

First, she identified the trigger—guilt-tripping about family time—and set realistic expectations, acknowledging that her mother wasn't going to suddenly stop wanting more family time. She prioritized addressing this issue because of its significant impact on her well-being.

Amy chose a calm moment to have a conversation with Linda. Using "I" statements, she expressed her feelings: "Mom, I love spending time with the family, but I feel stressed when I'm made to feel guilty about my time. I want to find a balance that works for both of us."

She then proposed a specific plan: "How about we schedule a weekly phone call and plan one big family gathering each season? This way, we stay connected regularly, and I can also manage my other commitments."

By communicating clearly and offering a solution, Amy was able to reduce conflict and establish a more sustainable arrangement.

Case Study 2: The Career Critique

Mike's father, Tom, constantly criticized Mike's career choices. Every conversation seemed to circle back to why Mike should have become a doctor instead of a teacher.

Mike decided to employ the emotional distancing technique known as the Observer. During their next interaction, when Tom started his usual criticism, Mike imagined himself as an anthropologist studying an interesting cultural phenomenon.

This perspective helped Mike respond calmly: "I understand you want the best for me, Dad. I've chosen teaching because it aligns with my values and brings me fulfillment. While I appreciate your concern, I'm not open to discussing career changes."

Mike then redirected the conversation to a topic they both enjoyed— their shared love of baseball. By setting a clear boundary and shifting the focus, Mike was able to have a more positive interaction with his father.

Case Study 3: The Unsolicited Advice Overload

Emma's mother, Janet, had a habit of offering unsolicited advice on everything from Emma's parenting style to her choice of curtains, making Emma feel constantly judged and undermined.

To address this, Emma decided to use the Sandwich Method. During a calm moment, she expressed her thoughts: "Mom, I know your advice comes from a place of love, and I appreciate that you want to help. However, I feel overwhelmed when I receive a lot of unsolicited advice. I value our relationship and would love it if we could focus on enjoying our time together instead of problem-solving."

Emma also set a clear boundary: "If I need advice, I promise I'll ask for it. Otherwise, can we agree to focus on other aspects of our lives?"

By acknowledging her mother's good intentions, expressing her feelings clearly, and setting a boundary, Emma was able to shift the dynamic of their relationship.

These case studies demonstrate how the strategies we've discussed can be applied in real-life situations. Remember, it may take time and practice to implement these techniques effectively, but the potential for improved relationships is worth the effort.

As we wrap up this chapter on choosing your battles, remember that you have the power to shape your interactions with your emotionally immature parents. By identifying triggers, setting priorities, communicating effectively, and maintaining emotional detachment, you can create a more peaceful and fulfilling relationship dynamic.

In Chapter 4, we'll delve deeper into the crucial skill of setting clear boundaries. After all, knowing which battles to fight is only half the equation—you also need to know how to effectively defend your emotional territory.

CHAPTER 3 TAKEAWAYS

- Choose your battles wisely when dealing with emotionally immature parents. Not every issue requires engagement or confrontation.
- Learn to identify triggers and patterns that lead to conflicts. Being aware of these can help you prepare and respond more effectively.
- Common triggers often include criticism of life choices, unsolicited advice, comparisons to others, guilt-tripping, dismissal of feelings, and invasion of privacy.
- Use preemptive conflict resolution strategies like redirecting conversations, acknowledging concerns and moving on, taking time-outs, practicing empathy, and setting clear boundaries.
- Set realistic expectations for change in your parents. Focus on improving your own responses rather than trying to completely change them.
- Prioritize issues worth addressing based on their impact on your life, frequency, potential for positive change, emotional cost, and whether they violate important boundaries.
- Communicate effectively without escalating conflicts by using "I" statements, choosing the right timing, staying calm, listening actively, and focusing on specific behaviors rather than character attacks.
- Practice emotional detachment techniques like mindfulness, the "observer" technique, and setting emotional boundaries to protect your well-being during challenging interactions.
- Remember that choosing your battles is not about winning arguments, but about preserving your emotional energy and fostering healthier relationships.

- Applying these strategies takes practice and patience. Be kind to yourself as you learn to navigate interactions with emotionally immature parents more effectively.

CHAPTER 4
SETTING CLEAR BOUNDARIES

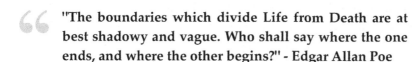 **"The boundaries which divide Life from Death are at best shadowy and vague. Who shall say where the one ends, and where the other begins?" - Edgar Allan Poe**

Boundaries are not walls; they are bridges that define where your responsibility ends and others' begins. Discover how setting clear boundaries can transform your relationship dynamics.

Now, I know what you might be thinking. "Silvia, isn't setting boundaries just a fancy way of pushing people away?" Trust me, I've been there. Growing up with a mother who could give a masterclass in emotional immaturity, I used to think boundaries were about erecting barriers. But I was mistaken. Boundaries are actually like bridges— they connect us to others in healthier, more authentic ways.

UNDERSTANDING BOUNDARY SETTING: THE WHAT, WHY, AND HOW

Alright, let's start with the basics. What exactly are personal boundaries? Think of them as your personal property lines. Just as you wouldn't want your neighbor to build a shed in your backyard without your permission, boundaries in relationships define what is and isn't acceptable.

I remember the first time I learned about boundaries. I was in my thirties, sitting in a therapist's office, overwhelmed by my mom's constant demands. The therapist asked me, "Silvia, what are your boundaries with your mother?" I stared at her blankly. Boundaries? With my mother? The concept was as foreign to me as speaking Klingon!

But here's the thing: boundaries aren't just for people with difficult relationships. They're for everyone. They're the secret sauce that makes relationships work. Why? Because they promote healthy relationships by:

1. Defining your limits: They help you communicate what you will and won't accept from others.

2. Protecting your well-being: They shield you from emotional manipulation and exhaustion.

3. Fostering respect: When others know your boundaries, they're more likely to respect them.

4. Enhancing self-esteem: Setting and maintaining boundaries shows that you value yourself.

Now, let's bust some myths about boundaries.:

1. **Myth: Boundaries push people away.**

Truth: Healthy boundaries actually bring people closer by creating clearer, more respectful relationships.

2. **Myth: Setting boundaries is mean.**

Truth: It's an act of self-care and respect for others.

3. **Myth: If you love someone, you shouldn't need boundaries.**

Truth: Love thrives when there are clear, respectful boundaries.

Remember, setting boundaries is a skill. Like any skill, it takes practice.

So be patient with yourself as you learn. It's okay to fumble a bit at first. Trust me, I've had my share of boundary-setting blunders!

TYPES OF BOUNDARIES: THE THREE MUSKETEERS OF PERSONAL SPACE

Now that we've got the basics down, let's talk about the different types of boundaries you can set. I like to think of them as the Three Musketeers of personal space: Emotional, Physical, and Time boundaries. All for one, and one for all!

1. Emotional Boundaries: The Heart Guards

Emotional boundaries are like the bouncers at the club of your heart. They decide who gets in and who stays out. With emotionally immature parents, these boundaries are crucial.

For example, I used to be my mom's emotional dumping ground. She'd call me at all hours, venting about her problems, leaving me drained and anxious. Setting an emotional boundary meant saying, "Mom, I care about you, but I'm not equipped to handle all your emotional needs. Let's talk about finding you a therapist."

Here are some ways to set emotional boundaries:

- Limit oversharing: It's okay to keep some things private.
- Avoid taking on others' emotions: You're not responsible for how others feel.
- Express your feelings: Use "I" statements to communicate your emotions.

2. Physical Boundaries: The Body Guards

Physical boundaries aren't just about personal space (though that's important too!). They're about respecting your body and your environment.

I remember when my mom used to barge into my room without knocking, even well into my adulthood. Setting a physical boundary meant saying, "Mom, please knock and wait for me to say it's okay before entering my room."

Physical boundaries can include:

- Personal space: How close you're comfortable with others being.
- Touch: What kind of physical contact you're okay with.
- Privacy: Respecting closed doors and personal belongings.

3. **Time Boundaries: The Clock Keepers**

Time boundaries are all about managing your availability and commitments. They're especially important with emotionally immature parents who might not respect your time.

For instance, my mom used to expect me to drop everything and rush over whenever she called. Setting a time boundary meant saying, "I can visit on Sundays between 2-4 pm. If it's an emergency outside those hours, please call 911."

Time boundaries can involve:

- Setting specific visiting hours
- Limiting the duration of phone calls
- Saying no to last-minute demands

Remember, these boundaries aren't about being rigid or unloving. They're about creating a structure that allows for healthier interactions. It's like creating a beautiful garden - you need fences to keep out the rabbits, but within those fences, beautiful relationships can grow!

TECHNIQUES FOR SETTING BOUNDARIES EFFECTIVELY: YOUR BOUNDARY-SETTING TOOLKIT

1. **Assertiveness Training: Finding Your Voice**

Being assertive is like being Goldilocks - not too passive, not too aggressive, but just right. It's about expressing your needs clearly and respectfully.

I used to be a people-pleaser extraordinaire. The thought of saying "no" to my mom made me break out in a cold sweat. But with practice, I learned to be assertive. Here's a simple formula I use:

- State the facts
- Express your feelings
- Make a specific request
- Explain the consequences

For example: "Mom, when you call me multiple times a day (facts), I feel overwhelmed and anxious (feelings). I need you to limit your calls to once a day unless it's an emergency (request). If you can't do this, I'll need to let your calls go to voicemail (consequences)."

2. Boundary Scripts: Your Go-To Phrases

Having a few ready-made scripts can be a lifesaver when you're put on the spot. Here are some of my favorites:

- "I understand you're upset, but I'm not comfortable discussing this right now."
- "I appreciate your input, but I've made my decision."
- "I need some time to think about that. I'll get back to you by [specific time]."
- "I'm not available right now, but I can talk on [specific day and time]."

Practice these in front of a mirror or with a friend. The more you use them, the more natural they'll feel.

3. Reinforcing Boundaries: The Art of Consistency

Setting boundaries is one thing; maintaining them is another. It's like planting a garden - you can't just plant the seeds and walk away. You need to water, weed, and tend to your boundaries regularly.

Here are some strategies for reinforcing your boundaries:

a) Be consistent: If you've set a boundary, stick to it. Inconsistency sends mixed messages.

b) Use positive reinforcement: Positive reinforcement isn't just for training pets; it's a powerful tool in human relationships too. When your parents respect a boundary, acknowledge it. A simple "I really appreciate you asking before dropping by" can go a long way. This approach encourages repeat behavior and helps create a more positive dynamic.

c) consistency is key. It's like tending a garden – you can't water it once and expect it to flourish. Regularly reinforcing your boundaries helps them take root and grow stronger over time. It might feel awkward at first, like you're wearing shoes that don't quite fit, but with practice, it becomes second nature.

Now, I know what you might be thinking—"Silvia, this all sounds great on paper, but what about when things get tough?" You're absolutely right. Setting and maintaining boundaries isn't always smooth sailing. There will be times when your emotionally immature parent pushes back, much like a toddler testing bedtime limits. This is where your resolve comes into play.

When faced with resistance, take a deep breath. Remind yourself why you set this boundary in the first place. It's not about punishing your parents; it's about taking care of yourself. Respond calmly but firmly, reiterating your boundary. You might say something like, "I understand you're upset, but I've made my decision and it's not up for discussion."

If the pushback continues, it's okay to disengage. You're not obligated to stand there and weather an emotional storm. A simple "I can see you're upset. Let's talk about this when we're both calmer," can work wonders. Then, follow through by stepping away if needed.

It's also crucial to have a support system in place. Whether it's a therapist, a support group, or trusted friends, having people who understand your journey can provide invaluable encouragement and perspective. They're like your personal cheerleading squad, reminding you of your strength when things get tough.

As you navigate this process, be patient with yourself. Rome wasn't built in a day, and neither are healthy boundaries. There might be times when you slip up or give in, and that's okay. It doesn't erase all the progress you've made. Dust yourself off, learn from the experience, and keep moving forward.

Remember, setting and maintaining boundaries is an act of self-care and self-respect. It's about creating a life that aligns with your values and needs. As you continue on this journey, you'll likely find that it extends beyond your relationship with your parents. The skills you're developing here can transform all areas of your life, from work relationships to romantic partnerships.

As we wrap up this chapter, take a moment to reflect on how far you've come. Setting boundaries with emotionally immature parents is no small feat. It takes courage, persistence, and a whole lot of self-love. Be proud of yourself for taking these steps toward a healthier, more balanced life.

In the next chapter, we'll delve deeper into the art of enforcing and adjusting boundaries. We'll explore how to adapt your boundaries as situations change, and how to handle those inevitable moments when boundaries are tested or crossed.

CHAPTER 4 TAKEAWAYS:

• Boundaries are not walls, but bridges that define where your responsibility ends and others' begins.

• Personal boundaries are essential for maintaining healthy relationships, especially with emotionally immature parents.

• There are three main types of boundaries:

- Emotional boundaries: Protect your emotional well-being

- Physical boundaries: Respect for your body and personal space

- Time boundaries: Manage your availability and commitments

• Setting boundaries is not selfish or mean; it's an act of self-care and respect for others.

• Assertiveness is key in communicating boundaries effectively. Use the formula: state facts, express feelings, make a specific request, and explain consequences.

• Having prepared scripts can help you set boundaries in challenging situations.

• Consistency is crucial in maintaining boundaries. Stick to your boundaries and use positive reinforcement when they're respected.

• Remember, setting and maintaining boundaries is a skill that improves with practice. Be patient with yourself as you learn.

• Healthy boundaries lead to healthier, more respectful relationships and improved self-esteem.

• While it may be challenging at first, especially with emotionally immature parents, setting clear boundaries is a powerful tool for personal growth and well-being.

CHAPTER 5

ENFORCING AND ADJUSTING BOUNDARIES

 "The boundary to what we can accept is the boundary to our freedom." - Tara Brach

S etting boundaries is a journey, not a destination. In this chapter, we'll explore how to effectively enforce and adjust boundaries to reclaim your personal space and emotional well-being.

As I've learned through my own healing from emotionally immature parents, setting boundaries is only the first step. The real challenge lies in consistently enforcing those boundaries and adjusting them as relationships evolve. It's a dynamic process that requires ongoing effort, self-awareness, and a willingness to adapt.

When we first begin setting boundaries with emotionally immature parents, it can feel like an uphill battle. We may face resistance, guilt-tripping, or even outright hostility. It's easy to get discouraged and revert to old patterns of people-pleasing or avoidance. But with the right strategies and support, we can learn to stand firm and create healthier relationships with both our parents and ourselves.

In this chapter, we'll explore the common challenges of boundary enforcement and how to navigate them with grace and resilience. We'll discuss practical techniques for reinforcing boundaries over time, even in the face of pushback or manipulation. Additionally, we'll dive into the art of adjusting boundaries as our relationships and needs evolve, helping us maintain autonomy and emotional well-being throughout our healing journey.

CHALLENGES IN BOUNDARY ENFORCEMENT

One of the biggest obstacles to maintaining boundaries with emotionally immature parents is the fear of conflict or rejection. We may worry that if we assert ourselves too strongly, we'll damage the relationship beyond repair. This fear is understandable, especially if we grew up in households where any expression of independence was met with disapproval or even punishment.

However, it's important to remember that healthy boundaries are not a rejection of our parents, but rather an affirmation of our own needs and desires. As Dr. Henry Cloud and Dr. John Townsend explain in their book Boundaries: When to Say Yes, How to Say No to Take Control of Your Life, "Boundaries define us. They define what is me and what is not me. A boundary shows me where I end and someone else begins, leading me to a sense of ownership."

In other words, boundaries are a way of taking responsibility for our own lives and well-being. They allow us to communicate clearly about what we will and won't tolerate in our relationships. While they may initially cause discomfort or pushback from our parents, in the long run, they are essential for building mutual respect and trust.

Another common challenge in boundary enforcement is navigating the guilt and emotional manipulation that often accompany standing up to emotionally immature parents. Our parents may try to make us feel selfish or ungrateful for asserting our needs or use fear and obligation to keep us in line. They might play the victim, resort to name-calling, or use criticism to wear down our resolve.

In these moments, it's crucial to remember that guilt is not a reliable indicator of whether we're doing the right thing. Just because someone feels hurt or angry about our boundaries doesn't mean those boundaries are wrong. In fact, as psychotherapist Amy Morin notes in her article 10 Ways to Build and Preserve Better Boundaries, "Feeling guilty doesn't mean you're doing something wrong. It's important to follow through with setting your boundaries, even if you feel guilty."

So how can we stay grounded in our boundaries, even when facing emotional manipulation? One key strategy is to practice self-valida-tion. This means learning to trust our own perceptions and feelings, rather than relying on others to define reality for us. We can remind ourselves that our needs and desires are valid, even if they aren't always convenient for others.

Another helpful technique is to use "I" statements when communi-cating our boundaries. Instead of accusing or blaming, we can calmly express how certain behaviors impact us. For example, instead of saying, "You're so controlling!" we might say, "I feel stressed when my decisions are questioned constantly." This approach keeps the focus on our own experience and helps avoid triggering defensiveness in others.

Of course, even with these strategies, we may still face resistance or pushback from our emotionally immature parents. They may refuse to respect our boundaries or escalate their behavior in an attempt to regain control. In such cases, it's important to have a plan for how to respond.

One option is to use the "broken record" technique—calmly repeating our boundary or request without getting drawn into arguments or justifications. For instance, if a parent repeatedly ignores our request not to comment on our weight, we can simply say, "I've asked you not to discuss my weight. Let's change the subject," each time the issue comes up.

Another strategy is to enlist the support of a neutral third party, such as a therapist or mediator, who can help facilitate difficult conversa-tions and keep everyone on track. Sometimes, having an outside perspective can make it easier for our parents to hear and respect our boundaries.

Ultimately, enforcing boundaries with emotionally immature parents requires a combination of inner work and outward communication. We need to be clear on our own needs and limits, practice asserting ourselves calmly and consistently, and be willing to follow through with consequences when necessary. It's not always easy, but with time and practice, it can become second nature.

TECHNIQUES FOR REINFORCING BOUNDARIES

Once we've set our initial boundaries with emotionally immature parents, the next challenge is to consistently reinforce them over time. This is where many of us struggle, as it's easy to slip back into old patterns or feel worn down by ongoing resistance. However, with the right techniques and support systems in place, we can learn to hold our ground and create lasting change in our relationships.

One of the most important factors in successful boundary reinforcement is consistency. As psychologist Dana Gionta explains in her article 10 Ways to Build and Preserve Better Boundaries, "Stick to your guns and don't vacillate. Boundaries that repeatedly cave in are not really boundaries at all." In other words, if we only enforce our boundaries sporadically or make exceptions when it's convenient, we send mixed messages that undermine our credibility.

To practice consistency, it helps to get clear on our non-negotiables— the boundaries we absolutely will not compromise on, no matter what. These might include things like physical or emotional safety, privacy, or autonomy in decision-making. By knowing our bottom lines ahead of time, we can respond more quickly and confidently when they are challenged.

Another key technique for reinforcing boundaries is to enlist the support of others. This could mean turning to friends, family members, or a therapist for validation and encouragement when we're feeling discouraged. It could also involve joining a support group or online community of others who are navigating similar challenges with emotionally immature parents.

Having a strong support network can make a huge difference in our ability to maintain boundaries over time. As researcher Brené Brown notes in her book *The Gifts of Imperfection*, "One of the greatest barriers to connection is the cultural importance we place on 'going it alone.' Somehow we've come to equate success with not needing anyone. Many of us are willing to extend a helping hand, but we're very reluctant to reach out for help when we need it ourselves... Until we can receive with an open heart, we're never really giving with an open heart."

In other words, asking for help is not a sign of weakness but of wisdom and strength. By surrounding ourselves with people who understand and support our boundaries, we create a powerful buffer against the negative influences of emotionally immature parents.

Even with a strong support system, maintaining boundaries can still be emotionally and mentally draining at times. That's why it's so important to prioritize self-care as part of our boundary reinforcement strategy. This means making time for activities that recharge and nourish us, whether it's exercise, meditation, creativity, or connecting with loved ones.

Self-care is not selfish—it's a necessary part of showing up fully in our relationships and responsibilities. As writer Anne Lamott puts it in her book Stitches: *A Handbook on Meaning, Hope, and Repair*, "Self-care is never a selfish act—it is only good stewardship of the only gift I have, the gift I was put on this earth to offer others. Anytime we can listen to our true self and give it the care it requires, we do so not only for ourselves, but for the many others whose lives we touch."

By filling our own cup first, we build the resilience and clarity needed to hold our boundaries with compassion and conviction. We teach others how to treat us by how we treat ourselves.

ADJUSTING BOUNDARIES AS RELATIONSHIPS EVOLVE

As much as we might wish for a "set it and forget it" approach to boundaries, the reality is that our relationships and needs are constantly evolving. What works for us at one stage of life may not feel right at another. That's why it's important to periodically reassess our boundaries and make adjustments as needed.

One common reason for boundary revisions is a change in life circumstances, such as getting married, having children, or starting a new job. These transitions can shift our priorities and reveal areas where our old boundaries no longer fit. For example, a new parent may need to set firmer boundaries around sleep schedules or family time, while someone starting a demanding job may need to limit their availability for social engagements.

Another catalyst for boundary adjustments is personal growth and healing. As we work through the pain and patterns of our past, we may find that our tolerance for certain behaviors or dynamics changes. We may become less willing to accept criticism or more assertive in expressing our needs. These shifts are a natural part of the healing process and a sign that we are developing a stronger sense of self.

Of course, adjusting boundaries with emotionally immature parents can be particularly tricky, as they may resist any changes that threaten their sense of control or entitlement. They may view our growth as a personal affront or try to undermine our progress by reverting to old manipulation tactics.

In these cases, it's important to approach boundary revisions with clarity and compassion. Start by getting clear on what specifically needs to change and why. Is there a particular behavior or dynamic that is no longer working for us? What would feel more supportive or respectful moving forward?

Once we have a sense of our goals, we can communicate them to our parents in a calm and direct way. It helps to frame the conversation around our own needs and feelings, rather than attacking or blaming.

For example, instead of saying, "You're so controlling!" we might say, "I've realized that I need more autonomy in my decision-making. Going forward, I'd appreciate it if you could trust me to handle things in my own way."

We can also offer specific examples of what the new boundary looks like in practice. If we're setting a boundary around unsolicited advice, we might say, "If I need help with a problem, I'll be sure to ask. But in general, I'd prefer to figure things out on my own first." By painting a clear picture of our expectations, we make it easier for our parents to understand and respect the new boundary.

Of course, even with the most tactful approach, our parents may still react negatively to boundary revisions. They may become defensive, dismissive, or try to argue us out of our position. In these moments, it's crucial to stay grounded in our own truth and not get hooked by their emotional volatility.

One way to do this is by using the "gray rock" method—a technique for communicating in a neutral, unresponsive way that gives difficult people little to react to. As author and blogger Shahida Arabi explains in her article How to Protect Yourself from Narcissists and Other Chronically Difficult People, "The gray rock method involves remaining as unresponsive and unreactive as possible, like a gray rock... The goal is to make yourself as boring, non-reactive, and uninteresting as a gray rock to the abusive person so that they will eventually lose interest in you."

In practice, this might involve calmly repeating our boundary without defending or explaining it, or ending conversations that veer into argument or disrespect. By refusing to engage in unproductive conflict, we send the message that our boundaries are non-negotiable and not up for debate.

Ultimately, adjusting boundaries is a skill that requires patience, persistence, and self-trust. It's normal to experience some trial and error as we figure out what works best for us and our unique family dynamics. The key is to stay anchored in our own worth and well-being, even when others resist or react.

As psychologist Ryan Howes notes in his article How to Set Boundaries with Difficult People, "Boundaries are the foundation of relationships, and the bedrock of self-care. Boundaries keep us safe from other people's actions, and perhaps even more importantly, from our own. Without boundaries, we can easily fall into other people's expectations for our lives, rather than fulfilling our own goals and needs."

By learning to set and adjust boundaries with emotionally immature parents, we reclaim our right to live a life that feels authentic and fulfilling. We begin to relate to our parents as autonomous adults, rather than obedient children. This shift invites healthier dynamics that can accommodate both our need for connection and our need for individuation.

In Chapter 6, we'll explore how adjusting our expectations of emotionally immature parents can help us find greater peace and acceptance on our healing journey. We'll discuss strategies for grieving the parent-child relationship we wish we'd had, while embracing the opportunity for self-parenting and reparenting. By learning to meet our own needs and validate our own feelings, we free ourselves from the endless pursuit of parental approval and step into our full potential.

CHAPTER 5 TAKEAWAYS

- Boundary enforcement is a dynamic, ongoing process that requires consistency, self-awareness, and adaptability.
- Common challenges in boundary enforcement include fear of conflict, guilt, and emotional manipulation from emotionally immature parents.
- Effective strategies for navigating these challenges include self-validation, using "I" statements, and enlisting the support of a neutral third party.
- Consistency is key in reinforcing boundaries over time, which means being clear on your non-negotiables and communicating them firmly and repeatedly.
- Building a strong support network of friends, family, or

professionals can provide validation and encouragement when enforcing boundaries feels challenging.

- Prioritizing self-care is essential for maintaining the emotional resilience and clarity needed to hold boundaries with compassion and conviction.
- As life circumstances and personal growth occur, it's important to periodically reassess and adjust boundaries to ensure they still align with your needs and values.
- When revising boundaries with emotionally immature parents, approach the conversation with clarity, compassion, and specific examples of what you need moving forward.
- The "gray rock" method can be a useful tool for communicating boundaries in a neutral, unresponsive way that gives difficult people little to react to.
- By learning to set and adjust healthy boundaries, you reclaim your right to a life that feels authentic and fulfilling, and invite your parents into a more Adult-to-Adult dynamic.

We are pleased to offer a FREE *Meditation Guide for Beginners*. Simply scan the QR code and follow the instructions to access your guide.
We hope it enhances your experience.

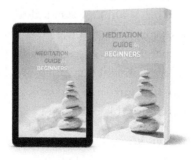

CHAPTER 6

ADJUSTING YOUR EXPECTATIONS

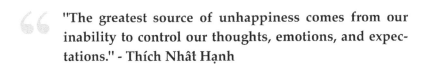 **"The greatest source of unhappiness comes from our inability to control our thoughts, emotions, and expectations." - Thích Nhất Hạnh**

Expectations shape our reality, but unrealistic expectations often lead to disappointment. Learn how adjusting your expectations can pave the way for inner peace and healthier relationships.

You're preparing for a family gathering, filled with a mix of hope and apprehension. Part of you imagines a picture-perfect event filled with laughter, heartfelt conversations, and a sense of true connection. Yet, deep down, you know this is unlikely when dealing with emotionally immature parents. As you walk through the door, your hopes are quickly dashed. Your parents are engaged in their usual patterns of bickering, criticism, and emotional unavailability. The disappointment feels like a punch to the gut, leaving you questioning why you continue to set yourself up for this pain.

If this resonates with you, know that you're not alone. As children of emotionally immature parents, we often find ourselves trapped in a cycle of unrealistic expectations and crushing disappointment. We cling to the hope that this time will be different, that our parents will finally provide the emotional support and stability we crave. But time and again, we're left feeling let down, hurt, and frustrated.

The hard truth is that holding onto unrealistic expectations is a surefire recipe for disappointment. It's like trying to plant a garden in concrete and expecting it to bloom. But here's the silver lining: by learning to adjust your expectations, you can break free from this painful cycle and cultivate inner peace and healthier relationships.

In this chapter, we'll take a deep dive into the art of managing expectations when dealing with emotionally immature parents. You'll gain insights into identifying unrealistic expectations, setting realistic ones, and developing the flexibility and resilience needed to navigate even the most challenging family dynamics.

IDENTIFYING UNREALISTIC EXPECTATIONS

The first step in adjusting our expectations is recognizing when they're unrealistic. This can be particularly challenging when we've grown up in an environment where emotional immaturity was the norm. Over time, we may have internalized the belief that if we just try harder, love more, or be better, our parents will finally give us the emotional support we need. But this belief, while understandable, sets us up for a cycle of disappointment.

Common pitfalls in expecting change from emotionally immature parents include:

1. **Believing that your love and efforts can "fix" them:** It's natural to want to help our parents grow and heal. However, it's crucial to understand that we cannot change our parents or make them emotionally mature. They must choose to embark on that journey themselves.
2. **Hoping that major life events will be a turning point:** We may think, "Surely, they'll rise to the occasion for my wedding/the birth of their grandchild/my college graduation." But emotionally immature parents often struggle

to show up in the ways we need, even during life's most significant milestones.

3. **Assuming that time will heal all wounds:** While time can provide perspective and growth opportunities, it doesn't automatically erase the impact of emotional immaturity. Without conscious effort and work, our parents are likely to fall back into old patterns.

Holding onto unrealistic expectations can take a heavy toll on our emotional well-being. Research published in the *Journal of Personality and Social Psychology* found that individuals with unrealistic expectations for their relationships report lower levels of satisfaction and higher rates of depression (Neff & Geers, 2013).

Similarly, a study in the *Journal of Social and Personal Relationships* showed that unmet expectations in family relationships are associated with increased feelings of loneliness and decreased life satisfaction (Deci et al., 2006).

So, how can we determine if our expectations are unrealistic? One helpful tool is the "Three C's" self-assessment:

The Three C's of Unrealistic Expectations:

1. **Control:** Do you believe you can control or change your parents' behavior?
2. **Cure:** Do you think your love and efforts can "cure" your parents' emotional immaturity?
3. **Consistency:** Do you expect your parents to consistently meet your emotional needs, despite a history of inconsistency?

If you answered "yes" to any of these questions, you might be harboring unrealistic expectations. But don't be discouraged - recognizing this is the first step towards positive change.

SETTING REALISTIC EXPECTATIONS

Now that we've identified unrealistic expectations, it's time to replace them with realistic ones. This doesn't mean settling for less or resigning yourself to a life of emotional neglect. Instead, it's about aligning your expectations with reality and focusing on what you can control - your own thoughts, feelings, and actions.

Here are some strategies for setting realistic expectations with emotionally immature parents:

1. **Accept their limitations:** Acknowledge that your parents are doing the best they can with the emotional tools they have. This doesn't excuse hurtful behavior, but it can help you approach interactions with compassion rather than frustration.
2. **Focus on your own growth:** Instead of trying to change your parents, direct your energy towards your own personal development. Seek therapy, read self-help books, attend workshops, and practice self-care.
3. **Find alternative sources of support:** Build a network of friends, mentors, and loved ones who can provide the emotional support and validation you may not receive from your parents. Surround yourself with people who uplift and inspire you.
4. **Communicate your needs clearly:** While you can't control your parents' reactions, you can express your needs and boundaries in a calm, assertive manner. Use "I" statements and focus on your own feelings rather than accusations. For example, "I feel hurt when you criticize my career choices. I need your support and encouragement."
5. **Prepare for their responses:** Anticipate that your parents may react with dismissiveness, defensiveness, or even aggression when you set boundaries. Have a plan in place for how you'll cope with these responses, such as deep breathing, walking away, or seeking support from a trusted friend.

One technique that can be particularly helpful is practicing acceptance without resignation. This means acknowledging reality without giving up on your own needs and desires. For example, you might say to yourself, "I accept that my parents may never be able to give me the unconditional love I crave, but I still deserve to be loved and supported. I can find that love and support elsewhere."

Grace, a 32-year-old teacher, had always hoped her emotionally immature mother would change. She would invite her mom to lunch, only to be met with criticism and coldness. After learning to set realistic expectations, Grace shifted her focus to her own growth. She started seeing a therapist, joined a support group for adult children of emotionally immature parents, and began practicing self-compassion. While her relationship with her mother remained challenging, Grace felt more at peace and empowered in her own life.

Another example is Mark, a 45-year-old entrepreneur who struggled with his father's lack of emotional support. Mark had always hoped his father would take an interest in his business ventures, but he was consistently met with indifference or criticism. By accepting his father's limitations and seeking mentorship elsewhere, Mark was able to build a thriving business and find fulfillment in his personal life.

By setting realistic expectations, we free ourselves from the constant cycle of hope and disappointment. We learn to find joy and fulfillment in our own lives, rather than waiting for our parents to change. Paradoxically, this can sometimes lead to improved relationships with our parents. When we stop trying to control or change them, we create space for more authentic, honest interactions.

CULTIVATING FLEXIBILITY AND RESILIENCE

Adjusting our expectations is an ongoing process, not a one-time event. As we navigate the ups and downs of relationships with emotionally immature parents, it's essential to cultivate flexibility and resilience.

Flexibility allows us to adapt to changing circumstances without getting thrown off course. It means being open to new ways of relating to our parents, even if they don't align with our ideal vision. For example, if your mother is consistently critical of your parenting style, you might set a boundary around discussing your children and instead focus on neutral topics like shared hobbies or current events.

Resilience, on the other hand, is the ability to bounce back from setbacks and disappointments. It's the inner strength that enables us to keep moving forward, even when our parents let us down or revert to old patterns. One way to build resilience is by practicing self-compassion. Rather than beating yourself up for having unrealistic expectations or getting upset when your parents disappoint you, try treating yourself with the same kindness and understanding you'd offer a close friend.

The American Psychological Association defines resilience as "the process of adapting well in the face of adversity, trauma, tragedy, threats, or significant sources of stress" (APA, 2014). Research has shown that resilience is not a fixed trait but a skill that can be developed and strengthened over time (Luthar et al., 2000).

Here are some other strategies for cultivating flexibility and resilience:

1. **Practice mindfulness:** Mindfulness helps us stay grounded in the present moment, rather than getting caught up in regrets about the past or worries about the future. Try taking a few deep breaths before interacting with your parents, and notice any thoughts or emotions that arise without judging them. Regular mindfulness meditation has been shown to reduce stress, anxiety, and depression (Goyal et al., 2014).
2. **Embrace humor:** Sometimes, laughter really is the best medicine. Try to find the humor in difficult situations, and don't be afraid to laugh at yourself. Humor can help us take ourselves less seriously and maintain perspective. Studies have found that humor and laughter can improve mood, reduce stress, and even boost immune function (Bennett & Lengacher, 2008).

3. **Keep a gratitude journal:** Each day, write down three things you're grateful for, no matter how small. This practice can help shift our focus from what's lacking to what's good in our lives. Gratitude has been linked to increased happiness, better sleep, and stronger relationships (Emmons & McCullough, 2003).

4. **Seek out new experiences:** Trying new things and stepping outside our comfort zones can help us build confidence and adaptability. Sign up for a class, travel somewhere new, or take on a challenging project at work. Engaging in novel experiences has been shown to promote brain plasticity and resilience (Kempermann et al., 2010).

5. **Surround yourself with positive influences:** Spend time with people who uplift and inspire you, whether that's friends, mentors, or role models. Their positive energy and support can help you weather even the toughest family storms. Research has consistently shown that strong social support is a key factor in resilience and well-being (Ozbay et al., 2007).

By cultivating flexibility and resilience, we become better equipped to handle whatever challenges come our way. We learn to bend without breaking, to find joy and meaning in life despite our parents' limitations. And in the process, we discover that we are stronger and more capable than we ever imagined.

Adjusting our expectations when dealing with emotionally immature parents is a process of letting go and embracing reality. It's about learning to accept our parents for who they are, while also honoring our own needs and boundaries. By setting realistic expectations, cultivating flexibility and resilience, and focusing on our own growth, we can break free from the cycle of disappointment and create more fulfilling lives.

Remember, you are not alone on this journey. There is a community of people who understand what you're going through and are here to support you. Reach out to trusted friends, family members, or a therapist when you need a listening ear or a shoulder to lean on.

As we move forward, let's explore the power of seeking support from trusted sources. In Chapter 7, we'll dive into the importance of building a strong support network and explore strategies for finding the guidance and encouragement needed to thrive.

Together, we can navigate the challenges of emotionally immature parents with grace, resilience, and self-compassion.

CHAPTER 6 TAKEAWAYS

- Holding onto unrealistic expectations of emotionally immature parents leads to a cycle of disappointment and emotional distress.
- Common unrealistic expectations include believing you can change your parents, hoping for a turning point, and assuming time will heal all wounds.
- Use the "Three C's" self-assessment (Control, Cure, Consistency) to identify unrealistic expectations.
- Set realistic expectations by accepting your parents' limitations, focusing on your own growth, finding alternative support, communicating clearly, and preparing for their responses.
- Practice acceptance without resignation by acknowledging reality while still honoring your own needs and desires.
- Cultivate flexibility by being open to new ways of relating to your parents and adapting to changing circumstances.
- Build resilience through mindfulness, humor, gratitude, seeking new experiences, and surrounding yourself with positive influences.
- Adjusting expectations is an ongoing process that requires letting go, embracing reality, and focusing on your own growth and well-being.
- You are not alone in this journey; seek support from trusted friends, family members, or a therapist when needed.

We are pleased to offer a FREE *Gratitude Journal*.
Simply scan the QR code and follow the instructions to access your
guide.
We hope it enhances your experience.

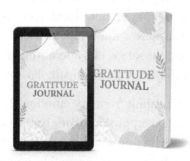

CHAPTER 7

BUILDING A SUPPORT SYSTEM: CRAFTING YOUR HEALING DREAM TEAM

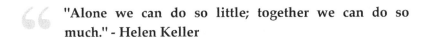 "Alone we can do so little; together we can do so much." - Helen Keller

No one can navigate the stormy seas of family dynamics alone. Discover the power of building a supportive network and seeking guidance from trusted sources during challenging times.

Have you ever felt like you're drowning in a sea of emotions, desperately trying to keep your head above water while dealing with emotionally immature parents? Trust me, I've been there. It's like being caught in a riptide—no matter how hard you swim, you just can't seem to break free. But here's the thing: you don't have to fight this battle alone. Trying to go it solo is like attempting to sail a ship through a storm without a crew. It's not just difficult; it's downright dangerous.

In my own journey of healing from my emotionally immature mother, I've learned that having a support network isn't just helpful—it's absolutely essential. It's like having a life raft in that stormy sea, keeping you afloat when the waves threaten to pull you under. In this chapter, we're going to explore how to build and leverage that support system, turning it into your personal lighthouse, guiding you through the fog of family dynamics.

Now, I know what some of you might be thinking. "But Silvia, I've always handled things on my own. Isn't asking for help a sign of weakness?" Let me stop you right there. Seeking support isn't a weakness; it's a strength. It takes courage to reach out, to be vulnerable, and to admit that you need help. And trust me, the rewards are worth it.

So, buckle up, because we're about to dive into the world of support networks. We'll explore different types of support, learn how to build and maintain these vital connections, and discover how to use them as a springboard for personal growth.

THE TYPES OF SUPPORT NETWORKS

When it comes to support networks, think of them as a buffet – there's something for everyone, and you can mix and match to create the perfect plate for your needs. Let's break down the main courses on offer:

Family, Friends, and Peer Support Groups

Family and friends can be your first line of defense. These are the people who know you best, who've seen you at your highest highs and lowest lows. When I first started grappling with the realization that my mother was emotionally immature, it was my best friend, Sophia, who listened to me rant for hours, offering tissues and chocolate as needed.

But here's a caveat—choose wisely. Not all family members or friends will understand your journey. Some may even be part of the problem, especially if they're enmeshed in the same dysfunctional family system. It's okay to be selective. Quality always trumps quantity.

Peer support groups are another goldmine of support. Imagine a room full of people who just get it. They've walked in your shoes, felt your pain, and now share their wisdom. It's like finding your tribe—your emotional home away from home.

I remember the first time I attended a support group for adult children of emotionally immature parents. The relief I felt was palpable.

Finally, I didn't have to explain or justify my feelings. These strangers understood me in a way even my closest friends couldn't. It was liberating.

Professional Support: Therapists and Counselors

These professionals are trained to guide you through the labyrinth of your emotions and experiences. Think of a therapist as your emotional personal trainer. Just as you'd hire a fitness trainer to help you get physically fit, a therapist helps you achieve emotional fitness. They provide tools, techniques, and insights that can significantly accelerate your healing process.

When I first started therapy, I was skeptical. How could talking to a stranger possibly help? But it was like someone turned on a light in a room I'd been fumbling around in the dark. My therapist helped me recognize patterns I'd never noticed, understand the root of my anxieties, and develop coping strategies I still use today.

Research supports this, too. A study published in the *Journal of Counseling Psychology* found that individuals who received counseling for issues related to family dysfunction showed significant improvements in their mental health and overall life satisfaction compared to those who didn't seek professional help.

Online Communities and Resources

Online communities and resources are like having a support group in your pocket, available 24/7. Forums, social media groups, and online workshops can offer a wealth of information and connection.

I'll never forget stumbling upon an online forum for adult children of narcissistic parents at 2 AM after a particularly difficult interaction with my mother. As I read through the posts, I felt a weight lift off my shoulders. These strangers on the internet understood my struggles in a way I had never experienced before.

However, a word of caution—the internet can be a double-edged sword. While it's a treasure trove of information and support, it's important to verify the credibility of sources and maintain healthy boundaries online. Not all advice is created equal, so it's crucial to balance online support with real-world connections.

Remember, the best support network is often a blend of different types. It's like creating a custom smoothie—you mix various ingredients to create the perfect combination for your taste and nutritional needs. In the same way, you can blend different types of support to build the ideal network for your emotional health and healing journey.

BUILDING AND MAINTAINING SUPPORT SYSTEMS

Alright, now that we've explored the different flavors of support available to us, it's time to roll up our sleeves and dive into the nitty-gritty of building and maintaining these lifelines. Think of this as your personal guide to constructing an emotional safety net that's strong enough to catch you when you're falling, yet flexible enough to grow with you.

Let's start with a truth bomb—not all support is created equal. Just as you wouldn't trust a rickety bridge to carry you across a chasm, you shouldn't rely on just anyone for emotional support. So, how do we separate the wheat from the chaff?

First, trust your gut. I know, it sounds cliché, but hear me out. Our intuition is often sharper than we give it credit for. If something feels off about a potential source of support—whether it's a therapist, a support group, or an online community—pay attention to that feeling.

When I was searching for a therapist, I met with three before finding the right fit. The first two were perfectly qualified on paper, but something just didn't click. The third? It was like talking to an old friend who happened to have a PhD in psychology. Don't be afraid to shop around until you find your perfect match.

Look for these green flags when identifying trustworthy sources of support:

1. They listen more than they talk.
2. They respect your boundaries.

3. They offer support without trying to "fix" you.
4. They have relevant experience or qualifications.
5. They're consistent and reliable.

Remember, it's okay to be picky. You're not just choosing a support system; you're choosing your healing companions. Make sure they're up for the journey.

Now that you've identified your support dream team, it's time to nurture these relationships. Think of this like tending a garden. You can't just plant the seeds and walk away – you need to water, weed, and care for your plants regularly.

Here are some techniques I've found invaluable:

1. Practice Active Listening: When someone in your support network is speaking, really listen. Put away your phone, make eye contact, and show that you're fully present. It's amazing how much deeper connections can grow when both parties feel truly heard.
2. Be Reliable: If you say you're going to call, call. If you commit to a support group meeting, show up. Consistency builds trust, and trust is the foundation of any strong support system.
3. Express Gratitude: Never underestimate the power of a heartfelt "thank you." Acknowledge the support you receive. It not only makes the other person feel appreciated but also reinforces the positive aspects of your relationship.
4. Offer Support in Return: Support should be a two-way street. Be there for your support network just as they're there for you. This reciprocity strengthens bonds and creates a sense of community.
5. Be Honest and Vulnerable: It can be scary to open up, especially if you've been hurt in the past. But allowing yourself to be vulnerable creates deeper, more meaningful connections.

I remember the first time I opened up to my friend group about my struggles with my mother. I was terrified they'd judge me or think less of me. Instead, their response was overwhelming support and love. That moment of vulnerability transformed our friendships into something deeper and more meaningful.

Setting Boundaries Within Support Networks

Now, here's where things get a bit tricky. It might seem counterintuitive, but setting boundaries within your support network is crucial. Why? Because even the most well-intentioned support can become overwhelming or unhelpful if not properly managed.

Think of boundaries as the fence around that garden we talked about earlier. They keep the good stuff in and the harmful stuff out. Here's how to set healthy boundaries:

1. Be Clear About Your Needs: Communicate what kind of support you need. Sometimes you might want advice, other times you just need someone to listen. Make your expectations clear.
2. Learn to Say No: It's okay to decline invitations or requests if you're not up for it. Your energy is precious, especially when you're healing.
3. Protect Your Privacy: You get to decide how much you share and with whom. Not everyone in your support network needs to know everything.
4. Manage Frequency of Contact: It's okay to limit how often you engage with your support network. Quality over quantity, remember?
5. Address Boundary Violations Promptly: If someone in your support network consistently oversteps, address it quickly and directly.

I learned this lesson the hard way when a well-meaning friend started calling me every day to "check in." While I appreciated her concern, it quickly became overwhelming. I had to gently explain that while I valued her support, daily calls were too much for me. Setting this boundary actually strengthened our friendship in the long run.

Remember, building and maintaining a support system is an ongoing process. It's okay if it feels awkward or challenging at first. Like any skill, it gets easier with practice. And trust me, the payoff is worth it. A strong, healthy support network can be the difference between merely surviving and truly thriving on your healing journey.

LEVERAGING SUPPORT FOR PERSONAL GROWTH

Picture your support network as a trampoline. Sure, it's there to catch you when you fall, but more importantly, it's designed to help you bounce back higher than before. That's the true power of a well-utilized support system – it doesn't just comfort you; it empowers you to grow.

Let's break down how this works:

1. Emotional Validation: When you share your experiences with your support network, you're likely to hear, "Your feelings are valid." This validation is incredibly healing. It helps counteract the gaslighting and dismissal you might have experienced from emotionally immature parents.
2. Different Perspectives: Your support network can offer fresh viewpoints on your situation. It's like they're holding up mirrors at different angles, helping you see aspects of yourself and your experiences that you might have missed.
3. Accountability: A good support system will gently hold you accountable for your healing journey. They're your cheerleaders, but they're also there to give you a loving nudge when you need it.
4. Safe Space for Practice: Your support network provides a safe environment to practice new behaviors and communication styles. It's like a dress rehearsal for real-life situations with your parents.
5. Stress Buffer: Research has shown that social support acts as a buffer against stress. A study published in the Journal of Personality and Social Psychology found that individuals with

strong social support experienced lower levels of stress
hormones when faced with challenging situations.

I remember when I first started setting boundaries with my mother. It was terrifying, and I was constantly second-guessing myself. But my support network was there, validating my decisions, offering advice, and most importantly, reminding me of my worth when I faltered. Their support didn't just help me heal; it made me more resilient.

CASE STUDIES HIGHLIGHTING SUCCESSFUL SUPPORT UTILIZATION

Now, let's bring this to life with some real-world examples. These aren't just success stories; they're roadmaps showing how others have leveraged their support networks to facilitate healing and growth.

Case Study 1: Laura, a 35-year-old teacher, grew up with an emotionally unavailable father and a mother who constantly criticized her. She joined a support group for adult children of emotionally immature parents and found it transformative.

"The group helped me realize I wasn't alone," Laura shared. "But more than that, it gave me a place to practice setting boundaries. I role-played difficult conversations with my parents before having them in real life. The feedback and support I received gave me the courage to finally stand up for myself."

Laura used her support group as a training ground, building confidence and skills she could apply in her relationship with her parents. This not only improved her family dynamics but also spilled over into other areas of her life, enhancing her self-esteem and professional relationships.

Case Study 2: Ethan, a 42-year-old accountant, struggled with anxiety and people-pleasing tendencies stemming from his relationship with his narcissistic mother. He decided to work with a therapist and joined an online support forum.

"My therapist helped me understand the root of my anxiety," Ethan explained. "But it was the online community that provided daily support and practical tips. Someone there suggested I start a 'victory journal' to document my small wins in setting boundaries. It was amazing to see my progress over time."

Ethan's case illustrates how professional and peer support can work in tandem. His therapist provided the tools, while his online community offered continuous encouragement and practical ideas.

These case studies show that successful support utilization isn't about leaning on others to solve your problems; it's about using your support network as a springboard for your own growth and healing.

Self-Help Resources and Tools for Ongoing Support

While your support network is invaluable, it's also crucial to develop tools for self-support. Think of these as your personal Swiss Army knife for emotional well-being. Here are some resources and tools I've found incredibly helpful:

1. Journaling: This is like having a conversation with yourself. It helps process emotions, track progress, and identify patterns in your thoughts and behaviors.
2. Meditation and Mindfulness Apps: Apps like Headspace or Calm can guide you through mindfulness exercises, helping you stay grounded during stressful times.
3. Self-Help Books: There are countless books on healing from emotionally immature parents. Some of my favorites include "Emotionally Immature Parents" by Lindsay C. Gibson and "Boundaries" by Henry Cloud and John Townsend. These books can provide insights and strategies when your support network isn't immediately available.
4. Podcasts: There are many great podcasts focused on mental health and healing from difficult family dynamics. They're like having a supportive voice in your ear during your commute or while doing chores.

5. Online Courses: Many therapists and counselors offer online courses on topics like setting boundaries, managing anxiety, or improving self-esteem. These can be a great way to supplement your healing journey.

6. Self-Care Toolkit: Create a personalized collection of activities, affirmations, and resources that help you feel grounded and calm. This might include favorite music, comforting scents, or inspiring quotes.

Remember, the goal is to build a diverse toolkit you can turn to in different situations. What works for you might be different from what works for someone else, and that's okay.

Now, here's a crucial point: these self-help tools aren't meant to replace your support network; instead, they work in tandem with it. Think of it this way—your support network is like a team of expert mountain climbers helping you scale the peak of healing. The self-help tools? They're your personal climbing gear. Both are essential for the journey.

I'll share a personal example. There was a time when I felt particularly overwhelmed by my mother's behavior, but it was late at night, and I didn't want to disturb my friends. I turned to my self-help toolkit. I did a guided meditation from my favorite app, wrote in my journal, and read a chapter from a self-help book. By the time I was done, I felt calmer and more centered. The next day, I was able to discuss the situation with my support group from a more grounded place.

As you build your self-help toolkit, remember to be patient with yourself. Healing isn't a linear process. There will be ups and downs, steps forward and steps back—that's normal and okay. The important thing is to keep going, keep learning, and keep growing.

One last thing before we wrap up this chapter: as you leverage your support network and self-help tools for personal growth, don't forget to celebrate your progress. It's easy to focus on how far we still have to go and overlook how far we've come. Take time to acknowledge your growth, no matter how small it might seem. Remember, every step forward is a victory.

In conclusion, building and leveraging a strong support network is a powerful tool in your healing journey. It provides validation, perspective, accountability, and a safe space for growth. Combined with self-help resources, it creates a robust system for ongoing healing and personal development.

As we move forward, remember that you're not just surviving; you're learning to thrive. You're not just healing; you're growing stronger. And you're not alone in this journey. Your support network, both people and tools, are there to help you every step of the way.

In Chapter 8, we'll explore another crucial skill in dealing with emotionally immature parents – the art of thinking and cooling down before you respond. This skill, when combined with a strong support system, can be a game-changer in your interactions with your parents. So, take a deep breath, give yourself a pat on the back for the work you've done so far, and let's continue this journey together.

CHAPTER 7 TAKEAWAYS:

- Support networks are essential: Healing from emotionally immature parents isn't a solo journey. A strong support system can be your lifeline in challenging times.
- Diversify your support: Combine family, friends, peer groups, professional help, and online communities for a well-rounded support network.
- Quality over quantity: Choose support sources wisely. Look for people who listen, respect boundaries, and offer consistent support.
- Nurture your connections: Practice active listening, be reliable, express gratitude, and offer reciprocal support to strengthen your relationships.
- Set healthy boundaries: Even within your support network, it's crucial to communicate your needs, learn to say no, and protect your privacy.
- Leverage support for growth: Use your network as a

trampoline for personal development. It can provide validation, fresh perspectives, and accountability.

- Develop self-help tools: Create a personal toolkit of resources like journaling, meditation apps, and self-help books to complement your support network.
- Celebrate progress: Remember to acknowledge your growth, no matter how small. Every step forward is a victory in your healing journey.
- Continual process: Building and leveraging a support network is an ongoing journey. Be patient with yourself and keep refining your support system as you grow.
- Prepare for the next step: A strong support network, combined with the skill of pausing before reacting, can transform your interactions with emotionally immature parents.

CHAPTER 8

THE PAUSE BUTTON: MASTERING MINDFUL RESPONSES TO DEFUSE EMOTIONAL LANDMINES

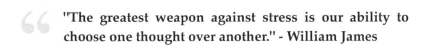 **"The greatest weapon against stress is our ability to choose one thought over another." - William James**

I n the heat of the moment, our reactions can define our relationships. Explore the art of mindful responding and how it can transform your interactions with emotionally immature parents.

Have you ever found yourself in a heated argument with your emotionally immature parent, only to walk away feeling drained, frustrated, and wishing you'd handled things differently? Trust me, I've been there more times than I can count. As someone who grew up with an emotionally immature mother, I know firsthand how challenging it can be to keep your cool when faced with triggering behavior. But over the years, I've learned that the key to transforming these interactions lies in mastering the art of mindful responding.

In this chapter, we'll explore the world of reactive behavior and dive into practical strategies for staying calm and collected, even in the face of emotional storms. I'll share the techniques that have been game-changers in my own journey, helping me navigate the treacherous waters of communication with my emotionally immature parents.

UNDERSTANDING REACTIVE BEHAVIOR: THE ROOT OF EMOTIONAL CHAOS

Let's start by peeling back the layers of reactive behavior. You know that moment when your parent says something that pushes all your buttons, and before you know it, you're firing back with words you'll later regret? That's reactive behavior in action, and it's like a runaway train—once it starts, it's hard to stop.

Psychological factors play a huge role in these impulsive reactions. Our brains are wired for survival, and when we feel threatened (even emotionally), our amygdala—the brain's alarm system—kicks into high gear. This triggers our fight-or-flight response, flooding our bodies with stress hormones like cortisol and adrenaline. In the blink of an eye, we're ready for battle, logic takes a backseat, and our emotional brain takes the wheel.

But here's the kicker: this lightning-fast response, while great for dodging predators in the wild, isn't so helpful when dealing with complex family dynamics. Studies have shown that when we're in this reactive state, our ability to think critically and empathize with others is significantly impaired (Arnsten, 2009). It's like trying to have a heart-to-heart conversation while running a marathon—not exactly ideal conditions for clear communication.

The consequences of reactive responses in communication can be significant. I remember a particularly heated argument I had with my mother over Thanksgiving dinner. She made a comment about my parenting style, and I exploded, accusing her of never being there for me as a child. The look of hurt on her face is something I'll never forget, and it took weeks to repair the damage caused by those few impulsive words.

Reactive communication often leads to:

- Escalation of conflicts
- Damage to relationships

- Increased stress and anxiety
- Missed opportunities for understanding and connection
- Reinforcement of negative patterns

But don't worry, all hope isn't lost! The first step in breaking free from reactive behavior is learning to recognize your triggers and impulses. This self-awareness is like having a secret superpower – it gives you the chance to pause and choose your response, rather than being at the mercy of your knee-jerk reactions.

One technique I've found incredibly helpful is keeping a "trigger journal." Every time you have a charged interaction with your parent, jot down:

1. What happened (the trigger)
2. How you felt (physically and emotionally)
3. How you reacted
4. The outcome of the interaction

Over time, you'll start to see patterns emerge. Maybe you notice that you're particularly sensitive to comments about your career choices, or that you tend to shut down when your parent uses a certain tone of voice. This knowledge is power – it allows you to anticipate potential hot spots and prepare yourself mentally.

Another useful tool is the STOP technique:

- S: Stop what you're doing
- T: Take a breath
- O: Observe what's happening internally and externally
- P: Proceed mindfully

By practicing this simple technique regularly, you'll train your brain to create a tiny but crucial gap between stimulus and response. It's in this gap that the magic of mindful communication happens.

STRATEGIES FOR MINDFUL COMMUNICATION: THE ART OF RESPONSIVE DIALOGUE

Now that we've explored the pitfalls of reactive behavior, let's shift gears and talk about the transformative power of mindful communication. This isn't about suppressing your emotions or becoming a Zen master overnight. It's about learning to engage with your emotionally immature parent in a way that honors your feelings while promoting understanding and growth.

The benefits of pausing and reflecting before responding are immense. Research shows that even a brief pause can activate our prefrontal cortex—the part of the brain responsible for rational thinking and emotional regulation (Davidson et al., 2012). This allows us to respond from a place of wisdom rather than reactivity.

I'll never forget the time I put this into practice during a phone call with my mother. She started criticizing my career choice, a topic that usually sent me into a defensive tailspin. But this time, instead of immediately jumping to defend myself, I took a deep breath and counted to five. In that brief moment, I reminded myself that her criticism likely stemmed from her own fears and insecurities. When I finally spoke, my voice was calm, and I was able to acknowledge her concerns while still asserting my own choices. The conversation took a completely different turn, and for the first time in years, we had a genuine dialogue about our hopes and fears.

To enhance your self-awareness and cultivate mindfulness, try incorporating these exercises into your daily routine:

1. The Three-Minute Breathing Space:
2. Minute 1: Acknowledge your thoughts and feelings
3. Minute 2: Focus on your breath
4. Minute 3: Expand awareness to your whole body
5. The Body Scan:
6. Lie down or sit comfortably
7. Slowly bring attention to each part of your body, from toes to head

8. Notice any sensations without judgment
9. Mindful Walking:
10. Take a short walk, focusing on the sensation of your feet touching the ground
11. When your mind wanders, gently bring it back to the physical experience of walking.

These practices help train your brain to stay present and aware, even in challenging situations. The more you practice, the easier it becomes to access this mindful state when you need it most.

When it comes to communication techniques that promote calm and clarity, the DEAR MAN approach (from Dialectical Behavior Therapy) has been a game-changer for me:

- Describe the situation objectively
- Express your feelings and opinions about the situation
- Assert yourself by asking for what you want or saying no clearly
- Reinforce your position by explaining consequences
- Stay Mindful of your objectives
- Appear confident
- Negotiate and be willing to give to get

For example, instead of lashing out when my mother criticizes my parenting, I might say: "Mom, when you tell me I'm too lenient with my kids (Describe), I feel frustrated and undervalued as a parent (Express). I'd appreciate it if you could trust my parenting decisions (Assert). This would help us have a more positive relationship and make me more open to your advice when I ask for it (Reinforce)."

By using these techniques, you're not just avoiding conflict – you're actively creating opportunities for deeper understanding and connection.

PRACTICING EMOTIONAL REGULATION: TAMING THE INNER STORM

Now, let's tackle one of the biggest challenges in dealing with emotionally immature parents: managing our own intense emotions. It's completely normal to feel anger, frustration, or sadness in these interactions. The key is learning how to navigate these emotional waters without capsizing the boat of communication.

One of the most effective tools I've found for managing anger and frustration is the RAIN technique, developed by psychologist Tara Brach:

- Recognize what's happening
- Allow the experience to be there, just as it is
- Investigate with kindness
- Non-identification (realize the emotion is not your whole identity)

I remember using this technique during a particularly frustrating phone call with my mother. She was going on about how I never visit enough, despite the fact that I had just been there the week before. As I felt my anger rising, I mentally went through the RAIN steps:

1. I recognized that I was feeling angry and defensive.
2. Instead of trying to push the feeling away, I allowed it to be there.
3. I investigated the feeling with curiosity – where was I feeling it in my body? What thoughts were accompanying it?
4. Finally, I reminded myself that while I was feeling angry, I wasn't just my anger. This emotion was a temporary visitor, not my entire identity.

This process helped me respond calmly, acknowledging my mother's desire to see me more while also asserting my own boundaries.

Another powerful tool for emotional regulation is the use of "I" statements. Instead of saying "You always criticize me!" try "I feel hurt when my choices are criticized." This shifts the focus from blame to expressing your own experience, which is much less likely to trigger defensiveness in the other person.

When it comes to de-escalating conflict situations, the STOP technique we discussed earlier can be a lifesaver. Additionally, here are some quick strategies you can use in the heat of the moment:

1. Take a time-out: It's okay to say, "I need a moment to collect my thoughts. Can we pause this conversation for five minutes?"
2. Use empathy: Try to see the situation from your parent's perspective, even if you disagree.
3. Find common ground: Look for areas where you and your parent agree, no matter how small.
4. Use humor (appropriately): Sometimes, a well-timed joke can diffuse tension and remind both parties of your shared humanity.

Jane, a client of mine, had a difficult relationship with her emotionally immature father. During a family gathering, he began criticizing her career choices in front of everyone. Instead of reacting defensively as she usually would, Jane took a deep breath, using the STOP technique, and calmly said, "Dad, I understand you're concerned about my future" (empathy). "How about we discuss this privately later?" (de-escalation). She then changed the subject to a shared interest—their love of baseball. This approach not only prevented a public argument but also opened the door for a more constructive conversation later.

Remember, mastering these techniques takes time and practice. Be patient with yourself as you learn and grow. Each interaction is an opportunity to strengthen your emotional muscles and improve your communication skills.

As we wrap up this chapter, take a moment to reflect on how far you've come. Learning to respond mindfully instead of reacting impulsively is no small feat, especially when dealing with emotionally charged family dynamics. You're doing important work, not just for your relationship with your parent, but for your overall emotional well-being.

In Chapter 9, we'll explore another crucial aspect of healing from emotionally immature parents: embracing the fact that you are not the parent in this relationship. This shift in perspective can be incredibly liberating, opening up new possibilities for growth and self-discovery.

So, take a deep breath, give yourself a pat on the back for all you've learned, and let's continue this journey together.

CHAPTER 8 KEY TAKEAWAYS:

- Reactive behavior is rooted in our brain's survival instincts but can be detrimental to communication.
- Recognizing your triggers is the first step in breaking free from reactive patterns.
- Mindful communication involves pausing, reflecting, and choosing your response intentionally.
- Techniques like RAIN and DEAR MAN can help manage intense emotions and promote clearer communication.
- De-escalation strategies, including empathy and finding common ground, can transform conflict into opportunities for understanding.

Action Steps:

1. Start a "trigger journal" to identify your emotional hot spots.
2. Practice the Three-Minute Breathing Space exercise daily.
3. Next time you're in a challenging conversation with your parent, try using the DEAR MAN technique.
4. Experiment with the RAIN method when you feel strong emotions arising.
5. Share your experiences and insights in a supportive community or with a trusted friend.

As we move forward, remember that changing long-standing patterns takes time and patience. Be kind to yourself as you practice these new skills.

In our Chapter 9, we'll explore how to shift your perspective and embrace your true role in the parent-child relationship.

CHAPTER 9

YOU ARE NOT THE PARENT!

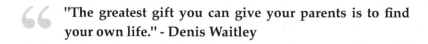 **"The greatest gift you can give your parents is to find your own life." - Denis Waitley**

B eing a caretaker in a parent-child relationship is natural. But what happens when the roles are reversed, and you find yourself parenting your own parents? Embrace your role as a child —it's not your burden to bear.

Have you ever felt like you're the adult in your relationship with your parents? Like you're constantly putting out fires, managing their emotions, or solving their problems? If so, you're not alone. I've been there, and let me tell you—it's exhausting. But here's the truth: it's not your job. You're not the parent in this relationship, and it's time to embrace that fact.

Growing up with emotionally immature parents, I often found myself in the caretaker role. I was the one soothing my mother's anxieties, mediating conflicts between my parents, and even managing our household finances. It felt natural at the time—after all, someone had to do it, right? Wrong. This role reversal, while it may seem necessary, can have profound impacts on our emotional well-being and personal growth.

In this chapter, we'll dive into the liberating truth that you are not—and should not be—your parents' caretaker. We'll explore how to recognize when you've been thrust into this role, the psychological toll it can take, and, most importantly, how to reclaim your rightful place as the child in your parent-child relationship. It's a journey of self-discovery and empowerment, and I'm here to guide you every step of the way.

So, buckle up. We're about to embark on a transformative journey that will help you shed the weight of inappropriate responsibilities and rediscover the freedom of being your parents' child, not their parent.

RECOGNIZING PARENTAL ROLE REVERSAL

Let's start by shining a spotlight on a phenomenon that's all too common in families with emotionally immature parents: role reversal. This is when children, whether young or adult, find themselves taking on parental responsibilities for their own parents. It's like a bizarre game of musical chairs where you end up sitting in the big chair, wondering how you got there and feeling like you don't quite fit.

Recognizing role reversal can be tricky, especially when it's been your normal for so long. Here are some telltale signs that you might be dealing with inappropriate parental expectations:

1. Emotional Caretaking: Are you constantly managing your parents' emotions? Do you find yourself walking on eggshells to avoid upsetting them, or spending hours on the phone listening to their problems? If so, you might be acting as their emotional caretaker.
2. Problem-Solving: Do your parents come to you with all their problems, expecting you to find solutions? Whether it's financial issues, relationship troubles, or work stress, if you're their go-to problem solver, that's a red flag.
3. Mediating Conflicts: If you often find yourself playing referee in your parents' arguments or smoothing over family disputes, you're taking on a parental role.

4. Financial Support: While it's normal to help out parents in genuine need, if you're regularly bailing them out financially or managing their money, that's stepping into parental territory.
5. Excessive Praise-Seeking: Do your parents constantly seek your approval or validation? This reversal of the normal parent-child dynamic is another sign of role reversal.

I remember when I first realized I was in this position. My mother had called me in tears over a disagreement with a neighbor. As I found myself brainstorming solutions and planning to intervene, it hit me: this wasn't my responsibility. I was acting more like a parent than a daughter.

Psychological Effects of Parental Role Reversal

1. Anxiety and Stress: Constantly worrying about your parents' well-being and feeling responsible for their happiness can lead to chronic anxiety. It's like carrying a backpack full of rocks everywhere you go - exhausting and overwhelming.
2. Delayed Personal Growth: When you're focused on parenting your parents, you might neglect your own growth and development. It's hard to spread your wings when you're always in the nest.
3. Difficulty in Relationships: The patterns you learn in your family can spill over into other relationships. You might find yourself always taking on a caretaker role, struggling to receive care from others, or having trouble setting boundaries.
4. Low Self-Esteem: Paradoxically, despite being "in charge," role reversal can lead to low self-esteem. You might feel like you're never doing enough or that your own needs aren't important.
5. Guilt and Resentment: It's common to feel guilty for wanting your own life, but also to resent the responsibilities placed on you. This internal conflict can be emotionally draining.

A study published in the Journal of Family Psychology found that parentification (another term for role reversal) in childhood was associated with higher levels of anxiety and depression in adulthood (Hooper et al., 2011).

Another study in the Journal of Clinical Psychology linked role reversal to difficulties in forming secure attachments in adult relationships (Macfie et al., 2015).

How Boundary-Setting Restores Appropriate Roles

Now for the good news: you can change this dynamic. The key? Boundaries. Setting clear, firm boundaries can help restore the appropriate roles in your relationship with your parents.

Here's how boundary-setting can help:

1. Clarifies Responsibilities: By setting boundaries, you make it clear what you will and won't do. This helps redefine your role as a child, not a parent.
2. Promotes Independence: When you stop solving all their problems, your parents have the opportunity to develop their own problem-solving skills.
3. Reduces Emotional Burden: Clear boundaries can help you detach from your parents' emotions, reducing your stress and anxiety.
4. Encourages Personal Growth: With boundaries in place, you'll have more time and energy to focus on your own life and personal development.
5. Improves Relationship Quality: Paradoxically, setting boundaries often leads to healthier, more balanced relationships in the long run.

I remember the first time I set a firm boundary with my mother. She called me at work, upset about a fight with my father. Instead of dropping everything to solve the problem, I took a deep breath and said, "Mom, I'm sorry you're upset, but I can't discuss this right now. I'm at work. Can we talk about this later when I'm off?" It was hard, and yes, she was initially upset. But over time, as I consistently reinforced this boundary, our relationship actually improved. She learned to respect my time, and I felt less burdened.

Setting boundaries isn't always easy, especially with emotionally immature parents who may resist the change. But remember, it's not just okay to set boundaries—it's necessary for your well-being and for the health of your relationship with your parents.

RECLAIMING PERSONAL IDENTITY AND AGENCY

Now that we've shone a light on role reversal, it's time to focus on you. Yes, **YOU!** It's time to reclaim your personal identity and agency. This isn't about being selfish; it's about being true to yourself and your needs. Remember, you can't pour from an empty cup, and you certainly can't be there for others if you're not there for yourself first.

Strategies for Asserting Independence and Autonomy

Asserting your independence might feel like you're trying to push a boulder uphill, especially if you've been in the caretaker role for a long time. But trust me, it's worth the effort. Here are some strategies to help you reclaim your autonomy:

1. Set Clear Boundaries: We talked about this earlier, but it bears repeating. Be clear about what you will and won't do. For example, "Mom, I can't be your therapist, but I can help you find a professional to talk to."
2. Practice Saying No: It's a small word with big power. Start small if you need to, but practice saying no to requests that infringe on your time or emotional energy.
3. Pursue Your Own Interests: Make time for hobbies, friendships, and activities that are just for you. This isn't selfish; it's necessary for your well-being.
4. Make Your Own Decisions: Start making choices based on what you want, not what you think your parents want. This could be as simple as choosing where to go for dinner or as significant as deciding on a career path.

5. Limit Information Sharing: You don't need to tell your parents everything. It's okay to keep some parts of your life private.

I remember when I decided to move to a different city for a job opportunity. My mother was upset and tried to guilt me into staying. In the past, I might have given in. But this time, I stood firm. I told her, "Mom, I love you, but this is an important opportunity for me. I'm going to take it." It wasn't easy, but it was a crucial step in asserting my independence.

Now, let's talk about self-care. And no, I don't just mean bubble baths and face masks (although those can be nice too!). I'm talking about deep, meaningful self-care that nurtures your personal growth and well-being.

1. Prioritize Your Physical Health: Regular exercise, healthy eating, and good sleep habits aren't just good for your body; they're essential for your mental and emotional well-being too.
2. Practice Mindfulness: Mindfulness meditation can help you stay grounded in the present moment, rather than getting caught up in your parents' drama. Even just five minutes a day can make a difference.
3. Journaling: Writing down your thoughts and feelings can help you process emotions and gain clarity. It's like having a conversation with yourself.
4. Pursue Personal Goals: Set goals for yourself that are separate from your family obligations. Whether it's learning a new skill, advancing in your career, or traveling, having personal goals helps maintain your sense of self.
5. Seek Therapy: A good therapist can provide invaluable support as you navigate this journey. They can help you process your emotions, develop coping strategies, and work through any lingering issues from your upbringing.

Techniques for Releasing Guilt Associated with Self-Prioritization

Ah, guilt. That pesky feeling that creeps in when we start prioritizing ourselves. It's like an uninvited guest that overstays its welcome. But here's the thing: you don't have to let guilt control you. Here are some techniques to help you release that guilt:

1. Challenge Your Thoughts: When you feel guilty, ask yourself: "Is this thought rational? Am I really doing something wrong by taking care of myself?" Often, you'll find that the answer is no.
2. Reframe Self-Care: Instead of seeing self-care as selfish, reframe it as necessary maintenance. Just like a car needs regular oil changes to run smoothly, you need self-care to be at your best.
3. Practice Self-Compassion: Treat yourself with the same kindness you'd offer a good friend. Would you tell a friend they're selfish for having boundaries? Probably not!
4. Visualize Your Future Self: Imagine yourself in the future, having prioritized your needs. How does that version of you feel? Probably happier and healthier, right?
5. Acknowledge Your Parents' Feelings Without Taking Responsibility: It's okay to recognize that your parents might be upset by your newfound independence. But remember, their feelings are their responsibility, not yours.

I struggled with guilt for years when I started prioritizing myself. I remember feeling terrible when I couldn't attend a family event because of work commitments. But then I realized something important: by taking care of my career, I was actually in a better position to help my family in the long run. This realization helped me release some of that guilt and embrace my choices.

Research supports the importance of self-care and releasing guilt. A study in the *Journal of Clinical Psychology* found that self-compassion was associated with lower levels of anxiety and depression (Neff et al., 2007). Another study in the *Journal of Personality and Social Psychology* showed that guilt-proneness was linked to lower well-being and life satisfaction (Tangney et al., 2007).

Remember, reclaiming your identity and agency is a process. It won't happen overnight, and there might be setbacks along the way. But each step you take toward asserting your independence, caring for yourself, and releasing guilt is a step toward a healthier, happier you.

As we wrap up this section, I encourage you to reflect on your own journey. Where have you been holding back? Where can you start asserting your independence? What self-care practices can you incorporate into your life? Remember, you're not just your parents' child— you're your own person with your own needs, desires, and dreams. It's time to embrace that.

Now, let's move on to the final piece of the puzzle: building healthy parent-child dynamics. Are you ready to redefine your relationship with your parents on your own terms? Let's dive in.

BUILDING HEALTHY PARENT-CHILD DYNAMICS

We've talked about recognizing role reversal and reclaiming your identity. Now it's time for the grand finale: building healthy parent-child dynamics. This is where the rubber meets the road, where we take everything we've learned and put it into action to create a more balanced, fulfilling relationship with our parents.

How Role Clarity Enhances Relationship Dynamics

Let's start by talking about role clarity. When everyone knows their role and sticks to it, it's like a well-oiled machine - everything runs more smoothly. Here's how clear roles can enhance your relationship with your parents:

1. Reduced Conflict: When roles are clear, there's less room for misunderstanding and conflict. You know what to expect from each other, and that clarity can be incredibly freeing.
2. Improved Communication: Clear roles make it easier to communicate effectively. You can speak to each other as adults, without the baggage of misplaced expectations.

3. Increased Respect: When you're not trying to parent each other, it's easier to respect each other as individuals. This mutual respect can transform your relationship.

4. Better Boundaries: Clear roles make it easier to maintain healthy boundaries. You're not constantly questioning whether you should step in and help - you know where your responsibilities begin and end.

5. Personal Growth: When you're not busy trying to fill a parental role, you have more energy to focus on your own growth and development.

I remember when I first started establishing clear roles with my parents. It felt awkward at first, like we were all actors who had suddenly been handed a new script. But as we settled into our proper roles, something amazing happened. Our conversations became more genuine. We started to see each other as we really were, not as the roles we had been playing. It was like a breath of fresh air in our relationship.

Setting Mutual Expectations for Healthy Interaction

Now, let's talk about setting expectations. This is crucial for building healthy dynamics. Here's how to go about it:

1. Have an Open Conversation: Sit down with your parents and have an honest discussion about your relationship. Share your feelings and listen to theirs.

2. Define Roles Clearly: Be explicit about what you see as your role and what you see as theirs. For example, "As your adult child, I want to have a loving relationship with you, but I can't be responsible for solving your problems."

3. Establish Boundaries: Discuss what kinds of support and interaction are appropriate. For instance, "I'm happy to listen and offer emotional support, but I can't provide financial assistance."

4. Agree on Communication Norms: Decide how often you'll

communicate and through what means. Maybe you agree to a weekly phone call, but texts are for emergencies only.

5. Plan for Conflict: Discuss how you'll handle disagreements when they arise. Having a plan in place can make conflicts less scary and more manageable.

Remember, this isn't a one-time conversation. It's an ongoing process of adjusting and refining your relationship. Be patient with yourself and your parents as you navigate this new terrain.

CASE STUDIES ILLUSTRATING SUCCESSFUL ROLE REDEFINITION

Let's bring this all to life with some real-world examples. Here are a couple of case studies that illustrate successful role redefinition:

Case Study 1: Natasha and her Mother: Natasha, a 35-year-old marketing executive, had always been her mother's confidante and problem-solver. When her mother's anxiety worsened after a divorce, Natasha found herself spending hours on the phone each day, neglecting her own work and relationships. Recognizing the unhealthy dynamic, Natasha took action:

1. She set clear boundaries around phone calls, limiting them to specific times and durations.
2. She encouraged her mother to seek professional help, offering to help find a therapist but not to be the therapist herself.
3. Natasha started practicing self-care, including therapy for herself to work through her own emotions about the situation.

Over time, Natasha's mother learned to manage her anxiety more independently. Their relationship evolved into a more balanced one, with Natasha able to enjoy her role as a daughter rather than a caretaker.

Case Study 2: Steve, a 28-year-old teacher, had been managing his father's finances since he was in college. His father, an artist with little financial acumen, had come to rely entirely on Steve for budgeting, bill payments, and financial decisions. This dynamic was straining their relationship and causing Steve significant stress. Here's how Steve redefined their roles:

1. He had an honest conversation with his father about the toll this responsibility was taking on him.
2. Together, they hired a financial advisor to take over the management of his father's finances.
3. Steve taught his father some basic budgeting skills, empowering him to take more control of his day-to-day expenses.
4. They agreed on a monthly "check-in" where they would discuss finances briefly, but not delve into minutiae.

The result? Steve's stress levels decreased dramatically, and he was able to enjoy spending time with his father without the burden of financial responsibility. His father, though initially resistant, gained a sense of pride in managing some of his own finances.

These case studies illustrate that change is possible. It may not be easy, and it certainly won't happen overnight, but with patience, persistence, and clear communication, you can redefine your relationship with your parents in a healthier way.

In Chapter 10, we'll explore another crucial aspect of healing from emotionally immature parents: practicing empathy. While it might seem counterintuitive to empathize with parents who may have caused us pain, understanding their perspective can be a powerful tool in our healing journey.

CHAPTER 9 TAKEAWAYS:

- Role reversal with emotionally immature parents can have significant psychological impacts.
- Recognizing signs of inappropriate parental expectations is the first step towards change.

- Setting boundaries is crucial in restoring appropriate parent-child roles.
- Reclaiming your personal identity involves asserting independence and practicing self-care.
- Building healthy parent-child dynamics requires clear communication and mutual understanding.
- Change is possible, as illustrated by real-life case studies of successful role redefinition.

Remember, embracing your role as the child doesn't mean you can't have a mature, adult relationship with your parents. It simply means that you're not responsible for parenting them. By maintaining this perspective, you open the door to a more balanced, fulfilling relationship - one where you can truly enjoy being their child.

As we close this chapter, I encourage you to reflect on your own relationship with your parents. Where do you see opportunities for role clarification? What steps can you take to assert your independence and reclaim your identity? Remember, every small step counts. You've got this!

Now, let's turn our attention to the power of empathy in healing from emotionally immature parents. Are you ready to explore how understanding can lead to freedom?

CHAPTER 10
PRACTICING EMPATHY

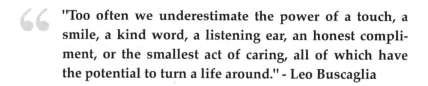 "Too often we underestimate the power of a touch, a smile, a kind word, a listening ear, an honest compliment, or the smallest act of caring, all of which have the potential to turn a life around." - Leo Buscaglia

Empathy bridges the gap between hearts, even in the most challenging relationships. Discover how practicing empathy can deepen understanding and foster connection with emotionally immature parents.

Have you ever felt like you're trapped in an emotional maze with your parents, constantly hitting dead ends and feeling frustrated? Trust me, I've been there. Growing up with my emotionally immature mother, I often felt like I was trying to communicate in a foreign language she couldn't understand. But here's the thing—empathy can be the universal translator we need in these challenging relationships.

Now, I can almost hear you thinking, "Silvia, are you seriously suggesting I try to empathize with the very people who've caused me so much pain?" Believe me, I get it. The idea of putting yourself in your parents' shoes might seem about as appealing as volunteering for a root canal without anesthesia. But stick with me here—empathy isn't about excusing their behavior or letting them off the hook. It's about understanding, and understanding is power.

In this chapter, we're going to dive deep into the world of empathy. We'll explore what it really means, how it differs from sympathy (yes, there's a significant difference!), and why it's such a game-changer when dealing with emotionally immature parents. I'll share some techniques that have worked wonders for me and my clients, and we'll look at how to apply empathy even in those hair-pulling, scream-into-a-pillow moments.

UNDERSTANDING EMPATHY: MORE THAN JUST WARM FUZZIES

Let's start with the basics. What exactly is empathy? It's not just a buzzword or something your yoga instructor talks about during savasana. Empathy is the ability to understand and share the feelings of another person. It's like having an emotional GPS that lets you navigate the inner landscape of someone else's heart and mind.

Now, here's where it gets interesting. Empathy isn't just one thing - it's actually a combination of three components:

1. Cognitive Empathy: This is the "I understand you" component. It's the ability to recognize and understand another person's emotional state. It's like being able to read the emotional weather forecast of someone else.
2. Emotional Empathy: This is the "I feel with you" part. It's when you can actually share the feelings of another person. Imagine it as having an emotional echo chamber in your heart that resonates with others' feelings.
3. Compassionate Empathy: This is the "I want to help you" element. It's when understanding and feeling lead to action. Think of it as the bridge between emotion and action.

Think of it like baking a cake. Cognitive empathy is your ingredients, emotional empathy is the mixing process, and compassionate empathy is putting it in the oven. You need all three to get the full, delicious result.

Now, let's clear up a common confusion: empathy is not the same as sympathy. Sympathy is feeling sorry for someone—it's standing on the shore, watching someone struggle in the water. Empathy, on the other hand, is jumping in with them. You're not just observing their struggle; you're trying to understand it from their perspective.

Here's a real-life example. When I was a teenager, my mom forgot my birthday. Again. With sympathy, I might have thought, "Poor me, my mom doesn't care." But with empathy, I tried to understand why. I remembered that her own mother had recently passed away, and she was struggling with depression. It didn't make it hurt less, but it helped me understand that her forgetfulness wasn't about me.

So why bother with all this empathy stuff, especially when it comes to emotionally immature parents? Well, the benefits are pretty impressive:

1. Better Communication: When you understand where someone's coming from, it's easier to find common ground. It's like having a universal translator for emotions. Imagine being able to decode the subtext behind your parent's words, understanding not just what they're saying, but why they're saying it.
2. Reduced Conflict: Empathy helps defuse tense situations. It's hard to stay angry at someone when you understand their perspective. It's like having a fire extinguisher for heated arguments.
3. Improved Emotional Intelligence: Practicing empathy makes you more attuned to emotions - both yours and others'. It's like upgrading your emotional software. You become better at recognizing and managing your own emotions, as well as understanding those of others.
4. Stronger Relationships: Empathy builds trust and deepens connections. It's the difference between a bridge and a wall.

When you show empathy, you're essentially telling the other person, "I see you, I hear you, and your feelings matter."

5. Personal Growth: Understanding others helps you understand yourself better. It's like holding up a mirror to your own emotions and experiences. As you practice empathy, you might find yourself gaining insights into your own behavior and reactions.

A study published in the *Journal of Counseling Psychology* found that individuals who practiced empathy in their relationships reported higher levels of relationship satisfaction and personal well-being (Cramer & Jowett, 2010). This research suggests that empathy isn't just good for your relationships—it's good for you, too.

Another fascinating study by Konrath et al. (2011) in the *Personality and Social Psychology Review* showed that empathy is associated with prosocial behavior, better mental health, and even improved physical health. Imagine that—by understanding others better, you could actually be boosting your own health!

But here's the thing: empathy isn't always easy, especially when it comes to emotionally immature parents. It's like trying to grow a garden in rocky soil. It takes effort, patience, and sometimes, a whole lot of emotional fertilizer. But the results can be truly transformative.

Remember, practicing empathy with emotionally immature parents doesn't mean you're letting them off the hook or excusing their behavior. It's not about saying, "It's okay that you forgot my birthday for the third year in a row." Instead, it's about thinking, "I wonder what's going on in your life that's making it hard for you to remember important dates." It's a tool for your healing, not theirs.

EMPATHY BOOT CAMP: TECHNIQUES FOR FLEXING YOUR EMPATHY MUSCLES

Alright, now that we've got the what and why of empathy down, let's roll up our sleeves and get into the how. Consider this your empathy boot camp. Don't worry, there won't be any push-ups involved (unless you want to do some – I hear they're great for stress relief). Instead, we're going to be working out our empathy muscles, and trust me, the results can be just as transformative as any physical workout.

Active Listening: It's Not Just Hearing, It's Understanding

First up, we've got active listening. This isn't just nodding along while you plan what you're going to say next. It's about truly tuning in to what the other person is saying – and what they're not saying. It's like being a detective, but instead of looking for clues at a crime scene, you're searching for clues in someone's words, tone, and body language.

Here's how to do it:

1. Give your full attention: Put away your phone, turn off the TV, and focus entirely on the person speaking. In our distraction-filled world, giving someone your undivided attention is like giving them a gift.
2. Use nonverbal cues: Maintain eye contact, nod, and use facial expressions to show you're engaged. Your body language can speak volumes about how attentive you are.
3. Don't interrupt: Let them finish their thoughts before you jump in. It's tempting to interject with your own thoughts or experiences, but resist the urge. Let them have the floor.
4. Reflect back: Summarize what you've heard to ensure you've understood correctly. "So what I'm hearing is..." This not only shows you're listening but also gives them a chance to clarify if you've misunderstood.
5. Ask open-ended questions: This shows you're interested and helps you understand more deeply. Instead of asking, "Did you have a good day?" try "How was your day?" The former can be answered with a simple yes or no, while the latter invites more detailed sharing.

I remember trying this with my mom when she was ranting about her coworkers. Instead of tuning out or arguing, I really listened. I asked questions like, "How did that make you feel?" and "What do you think led to that situation?" To my surprise, I realized her complaints weren't really about her coworkers – she was feeling undervalued and afraid of losing her job. It completely changed our conversation.

Perspective-Taking: Walk a Mile in Their Shoes (Even if They're Uncomfortable)

Next up is perspective-taking. This is where you mentally put yourself in the other person's position. It's like being an actor, but instead of memorizing lines, you're trying to understand someone's thoughts and feelings.

Here's a simple exercise:

1. Choose a situation where you and your parent disagreed.
2. Write down your perspective of what happened. Be as detailed as you can about your thoughts, feelings, and motivations.
3. Now, try to write about the same event from your parent's perspective. What were they thinking? Feeling? What motivated their actions? Remember, the goal isn't to justify their behavior, but to understand it.
4. Compare the two versions. What new insights do you gain?

I did this exercise after a fight I had with my mom over my career choice. From my perspective, she was being controlling and unsupportive. But when I tried to see it from her point of view, I realized she was scared. She grew up in poverty and was terrified I'd struggle financially. It didn't change her behavior, but it changed how I responded to it.

A study in the *Journal of Personality and Social Psychology* found that perspective-taking exercises like this one can increase empathy and reduce stereotyping (Galinsky & Moskowitz, 2000). It's like having a pair of empathy glasses that let you see the world through someone else's eyes.

Here's another perspective-taking exercise you can try:

The "Day in the Life" Exercise:

1. Choose a day when you had a difficult interaction with your parent.
2. Write down what you imagine their entire day might have been like, from the moment they woke up to when they went to bed.
3. Consider factors like their work stress, health issues, past experiences, and current worries.
4. Now, look at your interaction in the context of this imagined day. Does it change your perception of what happened?

Remember, the goal of these exercises isn't to excuse hurtful behavior, but to understand it. Understanding is the first step towards more constructive interactions.

Emotion Validation: You Don't Have to Agree to Understand

Last but not least, let's talk about emotion validation. This is acknowledging and accepting someone's feelings without necessarily agreeing with their actions or thoughts. It's like being a supportive friend who says, "I get why you feel that way," even if you don't think their feelings are justified.

Here's how to do it:

1. Identify the emotion: Try to name what the other person is feeling. Are they angry? Sad? Frustrated? Scared?
2. Acknowledge it: Let them know you see their emotion. "I can see you're really upset about this."
3. Normalize it: Show them their feeling is understandable. "It makes sense that you'd feel that way, given what you've been through."
4. Don't try to fix it: Resist the urge to immediately offer solutions or argue. Sometimes, people just need to feel heard.

I used this technique when my dad was angry about a political issue I disagreed with. Instead of arguing, I said, "I can see this really frustrates you. It must be upsetting to feel like your values are being ignored." He calmed down almost immediately, and we were able to have a real conversation.

Remember, validating doesn't mean agreeing. You're not saying, "You're right to feel that way," but rather, "I understand why you feel that way." It's a subtle but important difference.

A study in the *Journal of Marital and Family Therapy* found that emotion validation was associated with better relationship outcomes and individual well-being (Fruzzetti & Iverson, 2004). It's like emotional first aid—it doesn't solve all problems, but it can prevent a lot of unnecessary pain.

Here's a step-by-step guide to practice emotion validation:

1. Listen carefully to what the person is saying.
2. Identify the underlying emotion (it might not be explicitly stated).
3. Reflect back the emotion you've identified: "It sounds like you're feeling..."
4. Validate the emotion: "It's understandable that you'd feel that way because..."
5. Show support: "I'm here for you" or "Thank you for sharing that with me."

These techniques might feel awkward at first. That's okay! Empathy is like a muscle – the more you use it, the stronger it gets. Start small, maybe with a less charged interaction, and work your way up. You might be surprised at how quickly you start to see changes in your interactions.

EMPATHY IN ACTION: NAVIGATING THE STORMY SEAS OF CHALLENGING SITUATIONS

Alright, deep breath. We've covered the theory, we've practiced the techniques, and now it's time for the big leagues. How do we use empathy when emotions are running high, when past hurts are screaming for attention, and when every fiber of your being just wants to yell, "You don't understand me!"?

Empathy as a Conflict Resolution Superpower

First things first: empathy is your secret weapon in conflict resolution. It's like having a fire extinguisher for heated arguments. When you approach a conflict with empathy, you're not just trying to win – you're trying to understand. And understanding is the first step to resolution.

Here's how it works:

1. Cool down: If you're in the heat of an argument, take a moment to breathe. It's hard to be empathetic when you're seeing red. Try counting to ten, or even excuse yourself for a few minutes if you need to.
2. Listen actively: Remember those active listening skills we talked about? Time to put them to work. Focus on what the other person is saying, not on formulating your response.
3. Validate emotions: Acknowledge their feelings, even if you disagree with their perspective. "I can see this is really important to you."
4. Share your perspective: Use "I" statements to express your own feelings without blaming. Instead of "You always criticize me," try "I feel hurt when my choices are questioned."
5. Find common ground: Look for shared goals or values. Even if you disagree on the details, you might both want what's best for the family, for example.

Let me share a personal example. My mom and I used to have epic battles about my love life. She'd criticize my choices, I'd feel judged, and we'd both end up hurt and angry. One day, instead of defending myself, I tried empathy.

I said, "Mom, it sounds like you're really worried about my happiness. Is that right?" She burst into tears and admitted she was terrified I'd end up in an unhappy relationship like she had. It was a breakthrough moment. We still disagree sometimes, but now we can talk about it without World War III breaking out in our living room.

Let's look at a couple more real-life scenarios where empathy can work wonders:

Case Study 1: **The Holiday Guilt Trip Scenario**: Your dad is laying on the guilt because you're not coming home for the holidays.

Empathetic Approach:

- Listen to his concerns without interrupting. Let him express his disappointment fully.
- Validate his feelings: "I can Validate his feelings: "I can hear how disappointed you are. Family gatherings must be really important to you."
- Share your perspective: "I'm feeling torn because I want to see you, but I also need to [your reason]. It's not an easy decision for me."
- Find a compromise: Maybe suggest an alternative date for a visit or a way to include him in your plans. "What if we planned a special visit next month, just the two of us?"

Remember, the goal isn't to cave in to guilt, but to understand the emotions behind it and find a solution that respects both your needs.

Case Study 2: **The Career Critic Scenario**: Your mom constantly criticizes your career choices.

Empathetic Approach:

- Ask questions to understand her concerns. "What worries you most about my career?"
- Reflect back what you're hearing: "It sounds like you're worried about my financial stability and future security."
- Share your feelings: "When you criticize my choices, I feel like you don't trust my judgment. That hurts because your opinion matters to me."

- Find common ground: "We both want me to be successful and happy. Can we talk about what that looks like for each of us?"

In both these cases, empathy doesn't magically solve the problem. But it opens up a space for understanding and dialogue that wasn't there before.

Self-Reflection: The Secret Ingredient

Now, empathy isn't just about understanding others. It's also about understanding yourself. Self-reflection is the secret sauce that makes empathy truly powerful.

Try this exercise:

1. Think of a recent conflict with your parent.
2. Write down your initial reaction and feelings.
3. Now, dig deeper. What fears or insecurities might be driving those feelings?
4. How might your own experiences or beliefs be influencing your perspective?
5. Can you find any parallels between your reactions and your parent's behavior?

I'll go first. When my mom criticizes my parenting, my initial reaction is anger and defensiveness. But when I reflect, I realize it triggers my deep-seated fear of not being a good enough mother. Recognizing that helps me respond from a place of self-awareness rather than knee-jerk emotion.

A study in the Journal of Research in Personality found that self-reflection is positively associated with empathy and prosocial behavior (Joireman, Parrott, & Hammersla, 2002). It's like cleaning your empathy glasses—the clearer your view of yourself, the clearer your view of others.

Empathy in Extreme Situations: When It Feels Impossible

Now, I know what some of you might be thinking. "Silvia, this all sounds great, but you don't know my parents. They're impossible!"

I hear you. Sometimes, empathy can feel not just difficult, but downright impossible. Maybe your parents are abusive, or their behavior is so toxic that every interaction leaves you feeling drained and hurt. In these cases, it's crucial to remember that empathy is a tool for your understanding and healing, not an obligation to endure harmful behavior.

Here are some strategies for practicing empathy in extreme situations:

1. Maintain emotional distance: You can try to understand someone's perspective without absorbing their emotions or tolerating abusive behavior.
2. Set firm boundaries: Empathy doesn't mean allowing others to treat you poorly. It's okay to limit contact or set strict rules for interaction if that's what you need to protect your well-being.
3. Practice self-empathy: Sometimes, the person who most needs your empathy is yourself. Acknowledge your own pain and struggles.
4. Seek professional help: A therapist can provide invaluable support in navigating difficult family dynamics and practicing empathy in a way that's healthy for you.

Remember, empathy is not about excusing bad behavior or subjecting yourself to harm. It's about understanding, and sometimes understanding means recognizing that a relationship is unhealthy and taking steps to protect yourself.

THE RIPPLE EFFECT OF EMPATHY

As we wrap up this chapter, I want to share something amazing about empathy—it has a ripple effect. When you practice empathy, you're not just changing your relationship with your parents, you're changing how you interact with the world.

Research published in the journal Social Cognitive and Affective Neuroscience found that empathy training actually changes brain activity, increasing activity in neural networks involved in understanding others (Klimecki et al., 2014). It's like you're rewiring your brain to be more understanding and compassionate.

And this doesn't just affect your family relationships. The empathy skills you're developing can improve your friendships, romantic relationships, and even your professional life. You might find yourself becoming a better listener, a more effective communicator, and a more compassionate person overall.

Here's the thing: practicing empathy doesn't mean you'll suddenly have a picture-perfect relationship with your emotionally immature parents. It's not a magic wand that erases all the hurt and frustration. But it is a powerful tool for understanding, reducing conflict, and, most importantly, for your own growth and healing.

As we conclude this chapter, remember: empathy is a practice. Some days it'll flow easily, and other days it'll feel impossible. That's okay. Be patient with yourself. Every attempt at empathy, no matter how small, is a step towards better understanding and healthier relationships.

Try to make empathy a daily practice. It could be as simple as:

- Taking a moment to consider why a coworker might be in a bad mood
- Trying to see a disagreement with a friend from their perspective
- Reflecting on why a stranger's behavior in traffic might have upset you

The more you practice, the more natural it becomes.

In Chapter 11, we'll explore another crucial aspect of this healing journey: recognizing that healing isn't a destination, but a lifelong process. We'll dive into strategies for sustaining your progress and embracing the ongoing nature of personal growth.

But for now, take a moment to pat yourself on the back. You've just added a powerful tool to your emotional toolkit. Use it wisely, and watch how it transforms your interactions and, most importantly, your own peace of mind.

CHAPTER 10 TAKEAWAYS:

- Empathy is a powerful tool for understanding and improving relationships with emotionally immature parents.
- Empathy consists of three components: cognitive empathy (understanding), emotional empathy (feeling), and compassionate empathy (action).
- Empathy differs from sympathy; it involves understanding someone's perspective rather than just feeling sorry for them.
- Practicing empathy can lead to better communication, reduced conflict, improved emotional intelligence, stronger relationships, and personal growth.
- Active listening is a key skill in empathy, involving full attention, nonverbal cues, reflection, and open-ended questions.
- Perspective-taking exercises can help you understand your parent's point of view, even in disagreements.
- Emotion validation acknowledges others' feelings without necessarily agreeing with their actions or thoughts.
- Empathy can be a powerful tool in conflict resolution, helping to defuse tense situations and find common ground.
- Self-reflection is crucial in developing empathy, helping you understand your own emotions and reactions.
- In extreme situations, maintaining emotional distance and setting firm boundaries while practicing empathy is important.
- Empathy has a ripple effect, potentially improving all your relationships and changing how you interact with the world.
- Empathy is an ongoing practice; be patient with yourself as you develop this skill.
- Remember that empathy is a tool for your understanding and healing, not an excuse for tolerating harmful behavior.

CHAPTER 11

RECOGNIZING THAT HEALING ISN'T AN END STATE

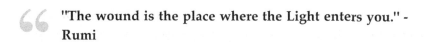 **"The wound is the place where the Light enters you." - Rumi**

Healing is not a destination but a journey—a journey of self-discovery and growth. Embrace the process and uncover the transformative power of continuous healing from parental emotional immaturity.

When we embark on the journey of healing from emotionally immature parents, it's natural to long for a definitive endpoint—that elusive moment when we can finally breathe a sigh of relief and declare ourselves completely healed. But as I've navigated my own path toward wholeness, I've come to realize that healing is less about reaching a finish line and more like tending to a garden. It's an ongoing process that requires patience, perseverance, and a willingness to embrace the inevitable ups and downs.

In this chapter, we'll explore why recognizing healing as a lifelong journey is not only realistic but also profoundly empowering. By shifting our perspective from "fixing" ourselves to nurturing our growth, we open the door to sustainable transformation and a deeper sense of self-acceptance.

EMBRACING THE JOURNEY OF HEALING

Picture a majestic oak tree, its branches reaching toward the sky and its roots delving deep into the earth. That tree didn't spring up overnight; it grew slowly and steadily, weathering storms and basking in sunshine, year after year. Our healing journey is much like the growth of that oak tree—a gradual, lifelong process that unfolds over time.

When we first acknowledge the impact of our emotionally immature parents, it's tempting to view healing as a one-time event, as if we could flip a switch and instantly undo years of emotional neglect or dysfunction. But as psychologist Dr. Margaret Paul explains, "Healing is not a linear process. It's a spiral. You keep coming back to things you thought you understood and seeing deeper truths."

This spiral nature of healing means that we may revisit the same issues or emotions at different stages of our lives, each time with a new level of understanding and self-awareness. For example, you might feel like you've made peace with your mother's inability to provide emotional support, only to find those old wounds resurfacing when you become a parent yourself. That doesn't mean you've failed in your healing—it means you're ready to explore a new layer of growth.

Research supports the idea that healing is an ongoing process. A study published in the *Journal of Counseling Psychology* found that individuals who experienced childhood emotional neglect continued to benefit from therapy and self-reflection well into adulthood, with new insights and coping strategies emerging over time (Davis et al., 2015). This suggests that our capacity for healing is not limited to a specific time-frame; rather, it's a lifelong journey of self-discovery and growth.

Common Challenges in the Healing Journey

Of course, embracing healing as a lifelong process doesn't mean it's always smooth sailing. Just like that oak tree weathering storms and droughts, we may encounter challenges and setbacks along the way. Some common obstacles in the healing journey include:

1. **Impatience and self-judgment**: When we're eager to feel better, it's easy to become frustrated with the pace of our progress. We may berate ourselves for not "getting over" our past faster or for still struggling with certain emotions or behaviors. But healing requires self-compassion, not self-flagellation. As researcher Dr. Kristin Neff notes, "Self-compassion involves treating ourselves kindly, like we would a good friend we cared about."

2. **Resistance to change**: As much as we may long for healing, part of us may also fear the unfamiliar territory of growth and transformation. We might cling to old patterns or defenses, even if they no longer serve us, simply because they're familiar. Psychotherapist Dr. Lissa Rankin compares this resistance to a caterpillar's metamorphosis: "The caterpillar doesn't resist the process of becoming a butterfly. It innately knows that the only way to access its true nature is to let go, surrender, and allow the transformation to unfold."

3. **Comparison and expectation**: In the age of social media, it's easy to fall into the trap of comparing our healing journey to others' highlight reels. We may see friends or acquaintances who seem to have it all together and wonder why we're still struggling. But healing is a highly individual process, and there's no one-size-fits-all timeline. As author Iyanla Vanzant wisely puts it, "Comparison is an act of violence against the self."

Recognizing these challenges as normal and even necessary parts of the healing process can help us approach them with greater self-compassion and resilience. Just like a seedling needs both sunshine and rain to grow, our healing journey requires both moments of ease and moments of discomfort.

How Acceptance Promotes Emotional Well-Being

One of the most powerful tools we have in navigating the lifelong journey of healing is acceptance. When we resist the reality of our past or the messiness of our present, we create additional suffering for ourselves. But when we learn to accept what is, we free up energy to focus on what we can change and cultivate greater emotional well-being.

Acceptance doesn't mean condoning hurtful behavior or resigning ourselves to unhappiness. Rather, it means acknowledging reality as it is, without judgment or resistance. As mindfulness teacher Dr. Jon Kabat-Zinn explains, "Acceptance is not passive. It is a courageous act of opening to life as it is, allowing what is to be what it is, and meeting it with mindfulness, compassion, and equanimity."

When we practice acceptance in the context of healing from emotionally immature parents, we allow ourselves to grieve the childhood we didn't have, to acknowledge the pain and hurt we experienced without getting stuck in resentment or bitterness. We learn to accept our parents' limitations—not as a way of excusing their behavior, but as a way of freeing ourselves from the expectation that they will change.

Research has shown that acceptance-based therapies, such as Acceptance and Commitment Therapy (ACT), can be highly effective in promoting emotional well-being and reducing symptoms of depression and anxiety (Kraemer et al., 2020). By learning to accept our thoughts and feelings without judgment, we create space for growth and transformation.

STRATEGIES FOR SUSTAINING PROGRESS

Self-Care Practices for Maintaining Emotional Health

As we navigate the lifelong journey of healing, self-care becomes a crucial component of sustaining progress and maintaining emotional health. Just as we need to nourish our bodies with healthy food and exercise, we need to nourish our hearts and minds with practices that promote resilience, self-compassion, and inner peace.

Some self-care practices that can support our healing journey include:

1. **Mindfulness and meditation**: Developing a regular mindfulness or meditation practice can help us cultivate

greater self-awareness, emotional regulation, and overall well-being. Research has shown that mindfulness-based interventions can be effective in reducing symptoms of depression, anxiety, and post-traumatic stress disorder (PTSD) (Khoury et al., 2013).

2. **Creative expression**: Engaging in creative activities, such as writing, art-making, or music, can be a powerful way to process emotions, express our authentic selves, and find meaning in our experiences. A study published in the Journal of the American Art Therapy Association found that art therapy can be an effective treatment for adults with a history of childhood trauma (Lobban, 2014).

3. **Connection and community**: Surrounding ourselves with supportive, understanding people can provide a vital source of validation, encouragement, and belonging. Joining a therapy group, attending workshops or retreats, or simply spending time with friends who "get it" can remind us that we're not alone in our healing journey.

Ultimately, self-care is about learning to treat ourselves with the kindness, compassion, and respect that we may not have received from our emotionally immature parents. It's about becoming our own loving inner parent and tending to our needs with gentleness and care.

Techniques for Managing Setbacks and Relapses

Even with a strong self-care practice, setbacks and relapses are a normal part of the healing process. We may find ourselves slipping back into old patterns, experiencing a resurgence of painful emotions, or feeling like we've lost ground in our growth. In these moments, it's important to remember that healing is not a linear journey, and setbacks don't define our overall progress.

Some techniques for managing setbacks and relapses include:

1. **Reframing setbacks as opportunities for growth**: Instead of viewing setbacks as failures, we can choose to see them as chances to deepen our self-awareness and strengthen our

coping skills. As author Brené Brown puts it, "Owning our story and loving ourselves through that process is the bravest thing that we will ever do."

2. **Practicing self-compassion**: When we're struggling, it's easy to fall into self-blame or self-criticism. But beating ourselves up only makes it harder to bounce back. Self-compassion involves treating ourselves with the same kindness and understanding we would offer a good friend. Research has shown that self-compassion is associated with greater emotional resilience, lower levels of depression and anxiety, and improved coping skills (Neff & Germer, 2013).

3. **Seeking support**: Setbacks can be isolating, but we don't have to face them alone. Reaching out to a therapist, support group, or trusted friend can provide a safe space to process our experiences and receive encouragement and guidance. Sometimes simply knowing that someone else understands and cares can make all the difference.

Building Resilience Through Ongoing Self-Reflection

One of the most powerful ways to build resilience is through ongoing self-reflection. By regularly taking time to check in with ourselves, process our experiences, and gain insight into our patterns and needs, we cultivate a deeper sense of self-awareness and self-trust. We learn to listen to our inner wisdom and make choices that align with our values and well-being.

Some self-reflection practices that can support resilience-building include:

1. **Journaling**: Writing about our experiences, thoughts, and emotions can be a powerful way to gain clarity, process difficult feelings, and track our growth over time. Research has shown that expressive writing can lead to improvements in physical and mental health, including reduced symptoms of depression and anxiety (Pennebaker & Smyth, 2016).

2. **Mindfulness**: Developing a regular mindfulness practice, such as meditation or yoga, can help us cultivate present-moment awareness, self-compassion, and emotional regulation. By learning to observe our thoughts and feelings without judgment, we create space for greater flexibility and resilience in the face of stress or adversity.

3. **Therapy or coaching**: Working with a therapist or coach can provide a structured space for self-reflection, skill-building, and growth. A skilled therapist can help us identify patterns, challenge limiting beliefs, and develop new coping strategies. They can also provide a safe, non-judgmental space to process difficult emotions and experiences.

CELEBRATING MILESTONES AND ACHIEVEMENTS

In the midst of the healing journey, it's easy to focus on how far we still have to go, rather than how far we've already come. But taking time to celebrate our milestones and achievements is a crucial part of sustaining motivation, building self-esteem, and recognizing our own strength and resilience.

When we acknowledge our personal growth, we remind ourselves that change is possible—that we are capable of overcoming challenges and creating a life aligned with our values and desires. We shift our focus from what's wrong to what's right, from our limitations to our potential. In doing so, we cultivate a sense of hope, pride, and self-compassion that fuels us forward on our healing path.

Some ways to celebrate milestones and achievements include:

1. **Keeping a success journal**: Writing down our accomplishments, breakthroughs, and moments of pride can help us track our progress and reflect on how far we've come. It can be especially powerful to look back on this journal during times of struggle or self-doubt.

2. **Sharing with supportive others**: Telling a trusted friend, family member, or therapist about our achievements can

provide a source of validation and encouragement. It can also help us feel less alone in our journey and more connected to a supportive community.

3. **Treating ourselves**: Celebrating milestones doesn't have to be grandiose or expensive. It can be as simple as taking a relaxing bath, buying ourselves a small gift, or enjoying a favorite meal. The key is to choose something that feels nurturing and honors our hard work and progress.

Setting Realistic Goals for Continuous Improvement

As we celebrate our achievements, it's also important to set realistic goals for continued growth and self-discovery. By breaking down our larger aspirations into smaller, manageable steps, we create a roadmap for ongoing healing and personal development.

When setting goals, it's important to remember the acronym SMART:

- **Specific**: Clearly define what you want to achieve, using concrete and measurable terms.
- **Measurable**: Identify how you will track your progress and know when you've reached your goal.
- **Achievable**: Choose goals that are challenging but realistic given your current resources and circumstances.
- **Relevant**: Ensure that your goals align with your values, needs, and overall vision for your life.
- **Time-bound**: Set a specific timeline for achieving your goal, with intermediate milestones along the way.

For example, instead of setting a vague goal like "be happier," you might set a SMART goal like "Practice gratitude by writing down three things I'm thankful for every day for the next month." This goal is specific (gratitude practice), measurable (daily for a month), achievable (simple and quick to do), relevant (cultivating positivity), and time-bound (one month).

By setting SMART goals, we create a sense of direction and purpose in our healing journey. We break down the sometimes overwhelming process of growth into bite-sized pieces, building momentum and confidence along the way. And as we achieve our goals, we reinforce the belief that we are capable of creating meaningful and lasting change in our lives.

CASE STUDIES

Throughout my years as a counselor, I've had the privilege of witnessing countless examples of resilience and perseverance in the face of childhood emotional neglect and immature parenting. These stories serve as powerful reminders that healing is possible, that we are not alone in our struggles, and that even the deepest wounds can be transformed into sources of strength and wisdom.

One such example is the story of Bianca, a woman in her mid-thirties who sought therapy to address the impact of her emotionally distant and critical mother. Bianca had spent years doubting herself, struggling with anxiety and perfectionism, and feeling like she was never good enough. Through therapy, she began to untangle the internalized messages from her mother and developed a stronger sense of self-worth and self-compassion.

Bianca's healing journey was not a straight line. There were times when she felt stuck, overwhelmed, or discouraged. But she remained committed to her growth, even in the face of setbacks and challenges. She practiced setting boundaries with her mother, even when it was uncomfortable. She learned to validate her own feelings and needs, rather than seeking approval from others. She surrounded herself with supportive friends and mentors who reflected back her inherent worth and potential.

Over time, Bianca began to see herself in a new light—not as a flawed or broken person, but as a resilient and capable woman who had survived a difficult childhood and was now thriving on her own terms. She started a successful business, formed healthy and fulfilling relationships, and became a mentor to other women who had experienced similar challenges. Her story is a testament to the power of perseverance, self-compassion, and the human capacity for growth and transformation.

Another example is Marcus, a man in his late twenties who grew up with an emotionally volatile and unpredictable father. Marcus had learned to walk on eggshells, never knowing when his father's mood would shift from jovial to rageful. As an adult, Marcus struggled with intimacy and trust in his relationships, often sabotaging connections out of fear of abandonment or rejection.

Through therapy and support groups, Marcus began to process the trauma of his childhood and learn new ways of relating to himself and others. He practiced vulnerability and assertiveness, learning to express his needs and desires in healthy ways. He worked on building self-esteem and self-compassion, challenging the belief that he was unlovable or undeserving of care.

Like Bianca, Marcus's healing journey was not without its ups and downs. He experienced moments of grief, anger, and despair as he confronted the pain of his past. But he also experienced moments of profound insight, connection, and joy as he began to build a life that aligned with his true self.

A turning point for Marcus came when he decided to pursue his life-long dream of becoming a writer. For years, he had been afraid to put himself out there, worried about judgment or rejection. But with the encouragement of his therapist and friends, he began to write and share his work with others. To his surprise, his writing resonated deeply with people, and he received positive feedback and recognition for his talent and vulnerability.

Through his writing, Marcus found a sense of purpose and meaning that had previously eluded him. He discovered that his painful experiences had also given him a unique perspective and depth of understanding, which he could use to help others. He became an advocate for mental health awareness and began to speak publicly about his own journey of healing and self-discovery.

Throughout this chapter, we've explored key strategies for sustaining progress and building resilience in the face of setbacks and challenges. We've discussed the importance of self-care, self-reflection, and celebration, and seen how these practices can lead to profound transformation and growth.

But perhaps most importantly, we've been reminded that healing is not something we have to do alone. By reaching out for support, sharing our stories, and connecting with others who have walked similar paths, we can find the validation, encouragement, and guidance we need to keep moving forward.

As we move forward, let's turn our attention to Chapter 12, where we'll explore the complex and often painful topic of estrangement from emotionally immature parents. While this may not be the path for everyone, for some of us, setting firm boundaries—or even cutting off contact—may be necessary for our own healing and well-being.

Remember, healing is a brave and beautiful choice, and you are worth every step of the journey. Keep shining your light, and know that you are never, ever alone.

CHAPTER 11 TAKEAWAYS

- Healing from emotionally immature parents is a lifelong journey, not a destination. Embracing the continuous nature of growth and self-discovery is key to sustainable progress and well-being.
- Common challenges in the healing journey include impatience, self-judgment, resistance to change, comparison, and unrealistic expectations. Recognizing these challenges as normal and even necessary parts of the process can help cultivate self-compassion and resilience.
- Acceptance is a powerful tool for promoting emotional well-being in the healing journey. By acknowledging reality without judgment or resistance, we free up energy to focus on what we can change and create space for growth and transformation.
- Self-care practices, such as mindfulness, creative expression, and connection with supportive communities, are crucial for maintaining emotional health and sustaining progress in the healing journey.

- Building resilience through ongoing self-reflection, including practices like journaling, mindfulness, and therapy, helps navigate the ups and downs of the healing process and cultivate inner resources for meeting life's challenges.
- Celebrating milestones and achievements, no matter how small, is essential for sustaining motivation, building self-esteem, and recognizing personal growth and resilience.
- Setting realistic goals using the SMART framework (Specific, Measurable, Achievable, Relevant, Time-bound) creates a roadmap for continued growth and personal development in the healing journey

CHAPTER 12
ESTRANGEMENT WHEN NECESSARY

 "The most courageous act is still to think for yourself. Aloud." - Coco Chanel

Sometimes, the bravest decision is to walk away. Explore the complexities of estrangement from emotionally immature parents and how it can be a pathway to reclaiming your mental and emotional health.

There comes a point in some people's lives when the only way forward is to boldly step away from those who have consistently hurt them, even if those people are family. It's a decision no one takes lightly, but it can be necessary for reclaiming your mental health, setting vital boundaries, and beginning the journey of self-discovery and healing. If you've been grappling with the complexities of potentially estranging yourself from your emotionally immature parents, know that you are not alone in this struggle.

In this chapter, we'll delve into the signs that estrangement may be necessary, strategies for navigating this incredibly difficult choice, and ways to cope with the aftermath.

SIGNS THAT ESTRANGEMENT MAY BE NECESSARY

Imagine living in a home where every day feels like navigating a minefield. You're constantly on edge, never knowing what might set off the next explosion of criticism, guilt-tripping, or emotional manipulation. You've tried to communicate your feelings countless times, but it's like shouting into a void. Your words are met with defensiveness, denial, or, worse, used against you in future arguments. If this scenario feels all too familiar, it may be a sign that your relationship with your emotionally immature parents has reached a breaking point.

But how do you know when it's truly time to consider estrangement? Here are some key indicators:

Toxic or Abusive Behavior

One of the most glaring red flags is a consistent pattern of toxic or abusive behavior from your parents. This can manifest in various ways, such as:

- Verbal abuse: Constant criticism, belittling, name-calling, or shaming
- Emotional abuse: Manipulation, gaslighting, guilt-tripping, or invalidating your feelings
- Physical abuse: Hitting, shoving, or any form of physical violence
- Sexual abuse: Inappropriate touching, sexual comments, or sexual assault

It's important to recognize that abuse doesn't always leave visible scars. Emotional and psychological wounds can be just as damaging, if not more so, because they can shape your self-perception and impact your relationships well into adulthood.

Emotional and Psychological Justifications

Even if your parents' behavior doesn't rise to the level of overt abuse, there may still be compelling emotional and psychological reasons to consider estrangement. For example:

- Your mental health is suffering: Interacting with your parents consistently leaves you feeling anxious, depressed, or emotionally drained. You find yourself dreading family gatherings or phone calls, and the negative effects linger long after the interaction ends.
- Your personal growth is stunted: Your parents' emotional immaturity and dysfunctional behavior patterns are holding you back from becoming the person you want to be. You feel trapped in old roles and dynamics that no longer serve you.
- Your other relationships are impacted: The stress and emotional turmoil from your parental relationship spills over into other areas of your life, causing strain on your friendships, romantic partnerships, or your own parenting.

A longitudinal study published in the Journal of Family Psychology found that adult children who experienced more parental rejection and invalidation in childhood reported greater psychological distress and lower self-esteem in adulthood (Rohner, 2004). This research highlights the long-term impact of emotionally immature parenting and the importance of prioritizing your own well-being.

Legal and Ethical Considerations

In some cases, estrangement may be necessary not only for your emotional well-being but also for legal or ethical reasons. For instance:

- Your parents engage in illegal activities: If your parents are involved in criminal behavior, such as substance abuse, theft, or fraud, you may need to distance yourself to avoid being implicated or enabling their actions.
- Your values and beliefs fundamentally clash: If your parents hold views or engage in behaviors that go against your core values, such as racism, homophobia, or religious extremism, you may feel compelled to take a stand by estranging yourself.
- Your children's safety is at risk: If you have children of your own and your parents' behavior puts them in physical or

emotional danger, your primary responsibility is to protect your kids, even if that means cutting off contact.

It's a heartbreaking reality that sometimes the people who are supposed to love and protect us end up being the ones who cause the most harm. However, recognizing that their behavior is unacceptable and taking steps to remove yourself from the situation can be an act of profound self-love and bravery.

STRATEGIES FOR SETTING BOUNDARIES IN ESTRANGED RELATIONSHIPS

So, you've weighed the signs and made the difficult decision to estrange yourself from your emotionally immature parents. Now what? Setting and maintaining boundaries is crucial for making this transition as healthy and stable as possible, both for yourself and for any other family members who may be impacted.

Communicating Your Boundaries

One of the most challenging aspects of estrangement is communicating your boundaries to your parents and others in your life. It's important to be clear, firm, and consistent in your messaging. Some tips:

- Be specific about what you need: Instead of making vague statements like "I need space," clearly define what that looks like for you. For example, "I won't be answering calls or texts for the next month while I focus on my mental health."
- Use "I" statements: Focus on expressing your own feelings and needs rather than accusing or blaming. For example, "I feel overwhelmed and need to step back from our relationship for my own well-being" instead of "You always make me feel terrible."
- Put it in writing: If a face-to-face conversation feels too daunting, consider writing a letter or email explaining your decision and boundaries. This allows you to carefully craft

your message and ensures there's a record of what was communicated.

A study published in the Journal of Social and Personal Relationships found that individuals who clearly communicated their boundaries and expectations in relationships reported higher levels of self-esteem and relationship satisfaction (Petronio, 2002). Remember, setting boundaries is not about punishing your parents; it's about taking care of yourself.

Managing Guilt and Societal Pressure

One of the biggest hurdles in estrangement is dealing with the guilt and societal pressure that often comes with "breaking up" with family. It's normal to feel a sense of obligation or to worry about the criticism and judgment you may face from others. However, it's crucial to prioritize your own well-being over the expectations of others.

Some strategies for managing these challenges:

- Reframe your perspective: Instead of viewing estrangement as a failure or a betrayal, try to see it as an act of self-care and a necessary step for your personal growth and healing.
- Surround yourself with support: Seek out friends, partners, or therapists who understand and validate your decision. Build a "chosen family" of people who have your back.
- Embrace your agency: Remember that you have the right to make decisions about who you allow into your life. No one is entitled to your time, energy, or forgiveness, family or not.

In a qualitative study of individuals who had estranged themselves from toxic family members, researchers found that many participants reported increased self-confidence, autonomy, and a sense of empowerment after setting boundaries (Scharp, 2019). It may feel scary and uncomfortable at first, but standing up for yourself can be incredibly liberating.

Estrangement is a complex and emotionally charged process, and it's essential to have access to resources and support along the way. Some options to consider:

- Therapy: Working with a licensed therapist who specializes in family issues can provide a safe space to process your emotions, develop coping strategies, and build resilience.
- Support groups: Joining an online or in-person support group for adult children estranged from their parents can offer a sense of community and validation. Hearing others' stories and sharing your own can be incredibly healing.
- Educational resources: Reading books, articles, or blogs about emotional immaturity, dysfunctional family dynamics, and estrangement can help you make sense of your experiences and feel less alone.

Remember, seeking help is not a sign of weakness; it's a testament to your strength and commitment to your own well-being. You don't have to navigate this difficult journey alone.

COPING WITH THE DECISION AND AFTERMATH

Making the decision to estrange yourself from your emotionally immature parents is only the beginning of the journey. The aftermath can bring up a host of complex emotions and challenges that require ongoing self-care and reflection.

Estrangement can be a rollercoaster of emotions, from relief and liberation to grief, anger, and everything in between. It's important to give yourself permission to feel the full range of your emotions without judgment. Some common experiences:

- Grief and loss: Even if your relationship with your parents was toxic, it's normal to mourn the loss of the parent-child bond you yearned for. Allow yourself to grieve the family you deserved but never had.

- Anger and resentment: As you process your experiences and set boundaries, you may feel a surge of anger towards your parents for their hurtful behavior. This is a valid emotion, but try to find healthy outlets for expressing it, such as journaling or physical activity.
- Guilt and self-doubt: It's common to second-guess your decision or feel guilty for "abandoning" your parents. Remind yourself that you are not responsible for their emotional well-being and that you deserve to prioritize your own healing.

A meta-analysis of studies on the psychological impact of estrangement found that individuals who had estranged themselves from toxic family members reported a mix of positive and negative emotions, with many experiencing a sense of loss alongside increased self-esteem and autonomy (Blake, 2017). Remember that healing is not a linear process, and it's okay to have mixed feelings.

Practicing Self-Care and Compassion

Estrangement can be emotionally and mentally exhausting, so it's crucial to prioritize self-care during this time. Some strategies to consider:

- Set aside time for activities that bring you joy and relaxation, such as reading, hobbies, or spending time in nature.
- Practice self-compassion by treating yourself with the same kindness and understanding you would offer a dear friend going through a tough time.
- Engage in regular exercise, healthy eating, and good sleep hygiene to support your physical and emotional well-being.
- Develop a mindfulness practice, such as meditation or deep breathing, to help manage stress and regulate your emotions.

Remember, taking care of yourself is not selfish; it's a necessary part of the healing process. You deserve to give yourself the love and nurturing that you may not have received from your parents.

Finding Hope and Healing

While estrangement can be an incredibly painful experience, it can also be a catalyst for profound personal growth and transformation. Many individuals who have gone through estrangement report a newfound sense of freedom, authenticity, and self-acceptance.

Consider the story of Jane, a 35-year-old teacher who distanced herself from her emotionally abusive parents after years of struggle. While the decision was heartbreaking, Jane found that the space and boundaries allowed her to flourish in ways she never thought possible. She developed healthier relationships, pursued her passions, and learned to trust her own instincts. "It was like taking off a heavy backpack that I had been carrying my whole life," Jane reflected. "I finally felt free to be my true self."

Jane's experience is not unique. A qualitative study of individuals who estranged themselves from toxic family members found that many participants reported increased resilience, self-efficacy, and post-traumatic growth following estrangement (Agllias, 2017). While the path is not easy, there is hope for healing and reclaiming your life on the other side.

As we close this chapter on estrangement, remember that this is not the end of your story—it is the beginning of a new chapter, one in which you get to be the author of your own narrative. In Chapter 13, we'll explore the power of acceptance in healing from emotionally immature parents, and how embracing the reality of your relationship can set you free.

CHAPTER 12 TAKEAWAYS: ESTRANGEMENT WHEN NECESSARY

- Estrangement from emotionally immature parents may be necessary for self-preservation and reclaiming mental and emotional health.
- Signs that estrangement may be necessary include toxic or abusive behavior, emotional and psychological distress, and legal or ethical concerns.

- Communicating boundaries clearly and consistently is crucial for navigating estranged relationships in a healthy way.
- Managing guilt and societal pressure can be challenging, but reframing your perspective, seeking support, and embracing your agency can help.
- Estrangement can bring up complex emotions like grief, anger, and self-doubt; allowing yourself to feel and process these emotions is an important part of healing.
- Prioritizing self-care and self-compassion is essential for coping with the aftermath of estrangement and supporting your overall well-being.
- While painful, estrangement can also be a catalyst for personal growth, increased resilience, and newfound freedom to be your authentic self.
- Accepting the reality of your relationship with your emotionally immature parents is a key step in the healing process and will be explored further in the next chapter.

CHAPTER 13

ACCEPTANCE OF THE ACTUAL RELATIONSHIP

"The first step toward change is awareness. The second step is acceptance." - Nathaniel Branden

A cceptance is not about condoning; it's about acknowledging reality and finding peace within it. Embrace the power of acceptance in your relationship with emotionally immature parents.

When I say "acceptance," I don't mean resignation or giving up on your hopes and dreams. Acceptance is about acknowledging reality for what it is, without judgment or wishful thinking. It's about making peace with the limitations and dynamics of your relationship with your parents, even if they're not what you want them to be. Acceptance doesn't mean condoning hurtful behavior or abandoning your boundaries. It simply means recognizing that you can't change your parents, but you can change how you react to and interact with them.

I know firsthand how difficult this can be. For years, I held onto the fantasy that my emotionally immature mother would suddenly transform into the nurturing, supportive parent I yearned for. I convinced myself that if I just tried harder, loved more, and tolerated more, she would finally give me the validation and unconditional love I craved. But the harder I tried, the more exhausted and resentful I became. It wasn't until I started practicing radical acceptance that I found the peace and emotional stability I had been searching for all along.

In this chapter, we'll explore the transformative effects of accepting the reality of your relationship with emotionally immature parents. We'll break down what acceptance really means, how it differs from resignation, and the benefits it can bring to your emotional well-being. We'll also dive into practical techniques for practicing acceptance, from mindfulness exercises to cognitive reframing strategies. And because acceptance isn't about abandoning your boundaries, we'll discuss how acceptance can actually enhance your ability to set and maintain healthy limits in your relationships.

UNDERSTANDING ACCEPTANCE IN RELATIONSHIPS

Before we dive into the details of how to practice acceptance, let's first define what we mean by acceptance in the context of relationships with emotionally immature parents. Acceptance is often misunderstood as resignation or giving up. People may think that accepting their parents' limitations means tolerating hurtful behavior or abandoning their own needs and desires. But that couldn't be further from the truth.

At its core, acceptance is about acknowledging reality without judgment. It's about seeing things as they are, not as we wish they were. When we practice acceptance in our relationships, we're not condoning bad behavior or lowering our standards. We're simply recognizing that we can't control or change other people, no matter how much we may want to. We acknowledge that our parents are who they are, with all their flaws and limitations, and that wishing for them to be different doesn't make it so.

Acceptance is also different from forgiveness, though the two concepts are often linked. Forgiveness is about releasing resentment and anger towards someone who has wronged us. It's a personal choice that can bring peace and freedom, but it doesn't necessarily require reconciliation. Acceptance, on the other hand, is about acknowledging the reality of a situation or relationship without necessarily forgiving the other person's actions. You can accept that your parent is emotionally immature and set boundaries accordingly, even if you haven't fully forgiven them for the pain they've caused you.

So why practice acceptance in relationships with emotionally immature parents? Because fighting reality is a losing battle. When we resist accepting the truth about our parents' limitations, we set ourselves up for constant disappointment and frustration. We expend precious energy trying to change someone who may not be capable of change, rather than focusing on our own growth and healing.

Acceptance, on the other hand, brings a sense of emotional peace and stability. When we stop fighting against reality and start working with it, we free up mental and emotional space for more positive pursuits. We can begin to set realistic expectations for our relationships rather than constantly being let down. We learn to detach from our parents' immaturity and focus on our own emotional well-being. Acceptance allows us to grieve the parent we never had while still appreciating any positive aspects of the relationship.

Of course, accepting the limitations of an emotionally immature parent doesn't mean we have to like those limitations. It's natural to feel sad, angry, or disappointed that our parents can't give us what we need. Acceptance isn't about suppressing those feelings, but rather acknowledging them without being ruled by them. It's about learning to coexist with difficult emotions rather than constantly struggling against them.

Practicing acceptance in relationships also opens up space for gratitude and appreciation. When we stop fixating on what our parents can't give us, we may start noticing the small ways in which they do show up for us. Maybe your mom can't provide emotional support, but she always remembers your birthday. Maybe your dad is quick to anger, but he also works hard to provide for the family. Accepting the full picture of our parents, flaws and all, allows us to develop a more realistic and balanced view of the relationship.

Benefits of Accepting the Actual Dynamics of Family Relationships

When we talk about accepting the actual dynamics of family relationships, we're acknowledging that every family has its own unique
patterns, roles, and ways of relating. These dynamics may be healthy
or unhealthy, but they are deeply ingrained and often resistant to
change. For those of us with emotionally immature parents, the family
dynamics may revolve around accommodating the parent's moods,
avoiding conflict, or playing certain roles to keep the peace.

Accepting the reality of these dynamics, rather than constantly fighting
against them, can bring significant benefits to our emotional well-
being. First and foremost, it can help reduce the constant stress and
anxiety that come from trying to change an unchangeable situation.
When we stop expending energy wishing our family were different,
we free up mental and emotional space for self-care, personal growth,
and more fulfilling relationships outside the family.

Acceptance can also help us establish healthy boundaries within the
family. When we acknowledge that our parents may never be able to
meet our emotional needs, we can start taking responsibility for
meeting those needs ourselves. We can learn to rely on ourselves and
other supportive people in our lives, rather than constantly seeking
approval or validation from our parents. Accepting the limitations of
the relationship allows us to adjust our expectations and communicate
our needs more clearly.

In addition, accepting the actual dynamics of the family can help us
develop greater compassion and understanding for our parents and
siblings. When we stop taking their behavior personally and start
seeing it as a product of their own unresolved issues and limitations,
we can develop a more objective perspective. This doesn't mean
excusing hurtful behavior, but rather understanding where it comes
from and setting boundaries accordingly.

Finally, accepting the reality of our family dynamics can be a crucial
step in breaking intergenerational cycles of emotional immaturity.
When we acknowledge the patterns that have been passed down
through the generations, we can start making conscious choices to do
things differently in our own lives. We can learn from our parents'

mistakes and strive to create healthier, more fulfilling relationships with our own partners and children.

TECHNIQUES FOR PRACTICING ACCEPTANCE

Mindfulness Exercises for Embracing Reality Without Judgment

One of the most effective tools for practicing acceptance is mindfulness. Mindfulness is the practice of being present and aware of your thoughts, feelings, and surroundings without judgment. It's about observing your experience without getting caught up in it or trying to change it. When we practice mindfulness in the context of relationships with emotionally immature parents, we learn to notice our reactions and emotions without being ruled by them.

Here are a few simple mindfulness exercises you can try:

1. **Breath awareness**: Take a few minutes each day to focus on your breath. Sit in a comfortable position and bring your attention to the sensation of air moving in and out of your nostrils. When your mind wanders (and it will), gently bring your attention back to your breath. This practice can help you cultivate a sense of calm and centeredness, even in the midst of difficult emotions.
2. **Body scan**: Lie down or sit in a comfortable position and bring your attention to your body, starting with your toes and moving up to the top of your head. Notice any sensations, tensions, or areas of relaxation. If you notice any discomfort or pain, simply acknowledge it without judgment and continue scanning. This practice can help you develop greater awareness of your physical and emotional state.
3. **Emotional labeling**: When you find yourself feeling a strong emotion in response to your parent's behavior, take a moment to simply name the emotion without judgment. For example, "I'm feeling angry right now" or "I'm feeling sad and disappointed." Labeling your emotions can help create a bit of

distance between you and the feeling, allowing you to respond rather than react.

4. **Loving-kindness meditation**: This practice involves silently repeating phrases of compassion and goodwill towards yourself and others. You can start by offering loving-kindness to yourself, then expand to include your emotionally immature parent, and eventually all beings. For example, you might say to yourself, "May I be happy. May I be healthy. May I be safe. May I live with ease." Then repeat the phrases for your parent and others.

Mindfulness takes practice, and it's normal for your mind to wander or for difficult emotions to arise. The key is to approach the practice with curiosity and self-compassion, rather than judgment or frustration. Over time, mindfulness can help you develop a greater capacity for acceptance and equanimity in the face of life's challenges.

Cognitive Reframing Techniques to Shift Perspectives

Another powerful tool for practicing acceptance is cognitive reframing. Cognitive reframing involves identifying and challenging unhelpful thoughts and beliefs, and replacing them with more balanced and realistic perspectives. When it comes to relationships with emotionally immature parents, we may have developed a number of cognitive distortions or unrealistic expectations that keep us stuck in cycles of frustration and resentment.

Here are a few common cognitive distortions and how to reframe them:

1. **All-or-nothing thinking**: This distortion involves seeing things in black and white, with no shades of gray. For example, you might believe that if your parent can't give you the emotional support you need, then they are a completely bad parent. Reframing this distortion might look like acknowledging that your parent has some positive qualities, even if they also have significant limitations.

2. **Mind reading**: This distortion involves assuming you know what someone else is thinking or feeling without direct evidence. For example, you might assume that your parent is intentionally trying to hurt you when they lash out, when in reality their behavior is more likely a result of their own unresolved issues. Reframing this distortion might involve reminding yourself that you can't know for sure what someone else is thinking, and focusing instead on how their behavior impacts you.

3. **Emotional reasoning**: This distortion involves assuming that your emotions reflect reality. For example, if you feel guilty for setting a boundary with your emotionally immature parent, you might assume that you are doing something wrong. Reframing this distortion might involve reminding yourself that feelings are not facts, and that it's okay to set boundaries even if it feels uncomfortable at first.

4. **"Should" statements**: This distortion involves holding yourself or others to unrealistic or rigid standards. For example, you might believe that your parent "should" be able to provide unconditional love and support, and feel resentful when they can't. Reframing this distortion might involve replacing "should" with "it would be nice if," and acknowledging that your parent may not be capable of meeting that ideal.

Cognitive reframing takes practice, and it can be helpful to work with a therapist or counselor to identify and challenge unhelpful thought patterns. With time and practice, reframing your thoughts can help you develop a more balanced and realistic perspective on your relationship with your emotionally immature parent.

Strategies for Letting Go of Unrealistic Expectations

One of the biggest barriers to accepting the reality of a relationship with an emotionally immature parent is holding onto unrealistic expectations. We may have grown up believing that if we just try hard enough, love enough, or tolerate enough, our parent will eventually give us the love and validation we crave. But the truth is, some people may never be capable of providing the emotional support and maturity we need, no matter how much we wish for it.

Letting go of these unrealistic expectations can be a painful and gradual process. It involves grieving the parent we never had and the relationship we may never have, while also learning to accept and appreciate the relationship for what it is.

Here are a few strategies for letting go of unrealistic expectations:

1. **Allow yourself to grieve**: Acknowledging and feeling the pain of not having the parent you needed is a crucial step in letting go of unrealistic expectations. Give yourself permission to feel sad, angry, or disappointed without judgment. You might find it helpful to write in a journal, talk to a therapist, or engage in a ritual to honor your grief.

2. **Identify your unmet needs**: Take some time to reflect on what emotional needs you were hoping your parent would meet, and how their inability to do so has impacted you. For example, you may have needed a parent who could validate your feelings, set consistent boundaries, or be emotionally present. Once you identify these unmet needs, you can start exploring alternative ways to meet them in your adult life.

3. **Adjust your expectations**: Rather than holding onto an idealized version of your parent, try to develop a more realistic view of their strengths and limitations. This might involve lowering your expectations for emotional intimacy or frequency of contact, while still appreciating any positive aspects of the relationship. Remember, accepting reality doesn't mean you have to like it; it simply means acknowledging what is.

4. **Practice self-compassion**: Letting go of unrealistic expectations can be a difficult and painful process. Be gentle with yourself as you navigate this transition, and remind yourself that you are doing the best you can with a challenging situation. Practice self-care activities that bring you comfort and joy, and

surround yourself with supportive people who can validate your experiences.

5. **Focus on your own growth**: Rather than fixating on what your parent can't give you, focus on your own personal growth and development. Set goals for yourself that are independent of your parent's approval or validation, and celebrate your own achievements and milestones. Remember, your worth and happiness are not contingent on your parent's ability to meet your needs.

Letting go of unrealistic expectations is a process, not a one-time event. It may involve setbacks, disappointments, and moments of grief. But with time and practice, releasing these expectations can bring a greater sense of peace and acceptance in your relationship with your emotionally immature parent.

BUILDING HEALTHY BOUNDARIES WITHIN ACCEPTED RELATIONSHIPS

Setting boundaries with emotionally immature parents can be challenging, as they may react with defensiveness, guilt-tripping, or emotional manipulation. However, approaching boundary-setting from a place of acceptance can actually make the process more effective and less stressful. Here's how:

1. **Clarity**: When we accept the reality of our parent's limitations, we can be more clear and specific in our boundary-setting. Rather than hoping our parent will intuitively understand our needs, we can communicate them directly and assertively. For example, instead of saying "I need you to be more supportive," we might say "I need you to respect my privacy and not comment on my weight."

2. **Consistency**: Accepting that our parent may never fully respect our boundaries can help us be more consistent in reinforcing them. Rather than getting caught up in cycles of hope and disappointment.

3. **Emotional detachment**: When we accept that our parent's behavior is not a reflection of our worth or lovability, we can set boundaries with less emotional reactivity. We can learn to detach from their immature responses and focus on our own well-being, rather than getting caught up in arguments or power struggles. This emotional detachment allows us to set boundaries from a place of clarity and self-respect.

4. **Realistic expectations**: Accepting our parent's limitations can help us set realistic expectations for their behavior and the relationship overall. We may not expect them to suddenly respect all our boundaries or meet all our needs, but we can expect them to face consequences if they consistently overstep. This shift in expectations can help reduce feelings of disappointment or frustration when boundaries are tested.

5. **Self-validation**: Perhaps most importantly, acceptance allows us to validate our own needs and feelings, rather than seeking validation from our emotionally immature parent. When we accept that our parent may never fully understand or support us, we can learn to trust and prioritize our own inner wisdom. We can set boundaries based on what we know is right for us, rather than what we think will please or appease our parent.

CASE EXAMPLES

Example 1: Setting Boundaries Around Unsolicited Advice

For years, I struggled with my mother's constant stream of unsolicited advice and criticism. No matter how I tried to communicate my needs or set limits, she always found a way to offer her opinion on my appearance, parenting choices, or career path. I would either react defensively or silently seethe with resentment, but nothing seemed to change.

It wasn't until I started practicing acceptance that I was able to set effective boundaries with her. I realized that her advice-giving was a deeply ingrained pattern, rooted in her own insecurities and need for control. I accepted that she might never fully understand how her behavior impacts me, no matter how clearly I communicate it.

With this acceptance, I approached boundary-setting with more clarity and less emotional reactivity. Instead of trying to convince my mother to change, I focused on setting clear, specific limits around her advice. For example, I might say, "Mom, I appreciate that you want to help, but I'm not looking for advice on this topic. If I need your opinion, I'll ask for it directly."

I also learned to end conversations or visits if my mother couldn't respect my boundaries. For example, if she started criticizing my appearance, I might say, "I've asked you not to comment on my weight. If you can't respect that, I'll need to end this conversation." Then, I would follow through, calmly and consistently.

Over time, my mother began to recognize that her unsolicited advice would be met with clear boundaries and consequences. Our relationship didn't magically transform, but I felt more empowered and grounded in my own choices. By accepting her limitations and focusing on what I could control, I was able to set boundaries with greater effectiveness and less stress.

Example 2: Navigating Holidays and Family Events

One of my clients, Tasha, always dreaded Christmas gatherings with her family. Her father would drink too much and pick fights, while her mother played the martyr, making passive-aggressive comments. Tasha often found herself in the role of peacemaker, trying to smooth things over and keep everyone happy.

Through our work together, Tasha began to practice acceptance around her family dynamics. She acknowledged that her parents were unlikely to change their behavior, no matter how much she wished for a "normal" family Christmas. She accepted that the gatherings would likely be stressful and triggering, and that she had limited control over her parents' actions.

With this acceptance, Tasha set clear boundaries for herself around the holidays. She decided to limit her visits to a few hours instead of staying overnight. She planned ahead for self-care activities, like taking walks or calling a supportive friend, to help cope with stress. She also practiced responses to common triggers, such as, "I don't feel comfortable discussing that topic" or "I need to step away for a moment to recharge."

Tasha communicated her boundaries clearly with her family ahead of time. She let them know she would be arriving and leaving at specific times, and that she wouldn't take on the role of mediator if conflicts arose. Instead of trying to control or change her parents' behavior, she focused on expressing her own needs and feelings.

While the holiday gatherings were still challenging, Tasha felt more grounded and empowered in her choices. By accepting the reality of her family dynamics and prioritizing her own well-being, she was able to navigate the events with greater peace and resilience.

SELF-ASSESSMENT TOOLS FOR MEASURING ACCEPTANCE AND GROWTH

As you practice acceptance and boundary-setting in your relationships with emotionally immature parents, it can be helpful to periodically assess your progress and growth. Self-assessment tools can provide insight into areas where you're thriving, as well as areas that may need more attention and support.

Here are a few self-assessment tools to consider:

1. **Emotional Maturity Scale**: This scale, developed by psychologist Sidney Jourard, measures emotional maturity across five dimensions: self-awareness, empathy, responsibility, flexibility, and integrity. By honestly assessing your own emotional maturity, you can identify areas for growth and celebrate your progress over time.
2. **Boundary Setting Self-Assessment**: This self-assessment, created by therapist Nancy Levin, helps you evaluate your boundary-setting skills across different areas of your life, including family relationships. The assessment includes

prompts like "I am able to say no without feeling guilty" and "I communicate my needs and wants clearly and directly." By reflecting on your responses, you can identify strengths and areas for improvement in your boundary-setting practice.

3. **Self-Compassion Scale**: Developed by researcher Kristin Neff, this scale measures your level of self-compassion across three dimensions: self-kindness, common humanity, and mindfulness. Practicing self-compassion is essential for navigating the challenges of relationships with emotionally immature parents, and this scale can help you track your progress over time.

4. **Personal Growth Initiative Scale**: This scale, created by psychologist Christine Robitschek, measures your motivation and skills for personal growth across four dimensions: readiness for change, planfulness, using resources, and intentional behavior. By assessing your personal growth initiative, you can identify areas where you may need more support or motivation in your journey towards acceptance and healing.

Throughout this chapter, we've explored the many facets of acceptance, from understanding its true meaning to incorporating it into our daily lives. We've discussed how acceptance differs from resignation or forgiveness, and how it can bring a greater sense of peace and emotional freedom in our relationships. We've also examined practical techniques for cultivating acceptance, from mindfulness practices and cognitive reframing to boundary-setting.

As you continue your journey of healing and growth, remember that you are not alone. There is a community of survivors and healers who understand your struggles and celebrate your triumphs. Seek out support when needed, whether from a therapist, support group, or trusted loved ones. Most importantly, never forget your inherent worth and lovability, no matter what your relationship with your parent may look like.

In Chapter 14, the final chapter, we will delve into the topic of forgiveness and how it fits into our healing journey. We'll explore what forgiveness really means, how it differs from acceptance, and how to practice it in a way that honors your boundaries and well-being.

CHAPTER 13 TAKEAWAYS

- Acceptance is not about condoning hurtful behavior or resigning yourself to a painful situation. It's about acknowledging reality as it is, without judgment or wishful thinking.
- Accepting the limitations and flaws of your emotionally immature parents can bring a greater sense of emotional peace, stability, and empowerment in your relationships.
- Practicing acceptance allows you to grieve the parent you never had while finding appreciation for the positive aspects of the relationship that do exist.
- Mindfulness techniques, such as breath awareness, emotional labeling, and loving-kindness meditation, can help you cultivate acceptance and reduce emotional reactivity.
- Cognitive reframing techniques, such as challenging all-or-nothing thinking and replacing "should" statements, can help you develop a more balanced perspective on your relationship with your parents.
- Letting go of unrealistic expectations for your parents is a process that involves grieving, self-compassion, and refocusing on your own needs and growth.
- Acceptance can enhance your ability to set clear, consistent, and effective boundaries with emotionally immature parents by reducing emotional reactivity and increasing self-validation.
- Seeking support from therapy, support groups, and additional resources is an important part of the ongoing journey of acceptance and healing.
- Remember that acceptance is a practice, not a destination. Be patient and compassionate with yourself as you navigate the challenges and rewards of this transformative process.

CHAPTER 14

FORGIVENESS FOR YOUR OWN SAKE

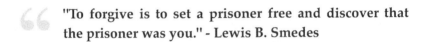 **"To forgive is to set a prisoner free and discover that the prisoner was you." - Lewis B. Smedes**

Hey there, fellow traveler on this journey of healing! Now, we're diving deep into the heart of forgiveness—not just any forgiveness, but the kind that sets your soul free.

When I first started my healing journey from my emotionally immature parents, forgiveness was the last thing on my mind. I mean, why should I forgive them? They were the ones who messed up, right? But as I've learned (and believe me, it was a rollercoaster), forgiveness isn't about letting them off the hook. It's about unhooking yourself from the pain of the past.

So, grab a cup of tea, get comfy, and let's explore this profound journey together. By the end of this chapter, you'll see forgiveness in a whole new light—as the ultimate act of self-love and liberation.

UNDERSTANDING FORGIVENESS: MORE THAN JUST SAYING "IT'S OKAY"

It's a crisp autumn morning, and I'm sitting in my favorite coffee shop, steam rising from my latte. Across from me is my friend Valerie, her eyes red-rimmed from crying. "I just can't forgive my mom," she says, her voice barely above a whisper. "If I forgive her, it's like saying what she did was okay."

Oh, Valerie. I felt that in my bones. Because that's exactly what I used to think forgiveness meant. But here's the kicker - that's not what forgiveness is at all.

So, what is forgiveness, really?

Forgiveness is a conscious, deliberate decision to release feelings of resentment or vengeance toward a person or group who has harmed you, regardless of whether they actually deserve your forgiveness. It's not about forgetting or condoning the hurt. It's about freeing yourself from the weight of anger and pain.

Now, let's break down the stages of forgiveness:

1. Hurt: This is where it all begins. You've been wounded, and the pain is real.
2. Anger: As a natural response to hurt, anger bubbles up. It's okay to feel angry!
3. Dialogue: This can be actual conversation with the person who hurt you, or an internal dialogue where you process your feelings.
4. Forgiveness: The decision to let go of resentment and negative feelings.
5. Release: Experiencing the freedom that comes with forgiveness.

Remember, this isn't always a linear process. You might bounce back and forth between stages, and that's perfectly normal.

Now, let's talk about why forgiveness is so good for you. And I'm not just pulling this out of thin air—there's solid science backing it up.

A study published in the *Journal of Health Psychology* found that forgiveness is positively associated with five key health measures: physical symptoms, medications used, sleep quality, fatigue, and somatic complaints. Participants who were more forgiving reported better health across all five areas (Lawler et al., 2005).

But wait, there's more! Forgiveness doesn't just improve your physical health—it's like a magic elixir for your mental well-being too. Research shows that forgiveness therapy can significantly reduce anxiety, depression, and perceived stress. It can even boost your self-esteem and sense of hope (Reed & Enright, 2006).

Now, I can almost hear you thinking, "But Silvia, if I forgive, doesn't that mean I have to reconcile with my parents?" And that, my friend, is where many people get tripped up. So let's clear this up once and for all:

Forgiveness is not reconciliation.

Let me say that again for the people in the back: **Forgiveness is NOT reconciliation**.

Forgiveness is an internal process—it's about changing your feelings and attitude toward the person who hurt you. Reconciliation, on the other hand, is about rebuilding a relationship. You can absolutely forgive someone without allowing them back into your life.

For example, I've forgiven my mother for her emotional immaturity and the pain it caused me. But that doesn't mean I've forgotten or allow her to continue hurting me. I've set clear boundaries (remember Chapter 4?), and while I've released the anger and resentment, I still protect myself from further harm.

Understanding this distinction was a game-changer for me. It allowed me to begin my forgiveness journey without the fear of having to subject myself to more hurt. And let me tell you, it was like taking off a backpack full of rocks I didn't even know I was carrying.

As we wrap up this section, I want you to remember: forgiveness is a gift you give yourself. It's not about the other person—it's about freeing yourself from the prison of resentment and pain. And trust me, the view from outside that prison? It's pretty spectacular.

Now, let's move on to something that might feel even trickier—forgiving ourselves. Because sometimes, the person we need to forgive most is staring right back at us in the mirror.

PRACTICING SELF-FORGIVENESS: BE YOUR OWN BEST FRIEND

It's 2 AM, and you're lying in bed, wide awake. Your mind feels like a hamster on a wheel, replaying every mistake, every "should have" and "could have" on an endless loop. Sound familiar? Yeah, I've been there too. This, my friends, is where self-forgiveness comes in.

Self-forgiveness is like being your own best friend. It's about treating yourself with the same kindness and understanding you'd offer someone you love. But let's be real—it's often easier said than done, especially when we've grown up with emotionally immature parents who may have constantly criticized us or made us feel like we weren't good enough.

So, how do we break free from this cycle of self-blame and guilt? Let's dive in.

First, we need to recognize that guilt and shame, while uncomfortable, can actually be helpful emotions when processed in a healthy way. Guilt tells us when we've done something that doesn't align with our values, while shame often stems from feeling like we are fundamentally flawed or unworthy.

The key is to listen to these emotions without letting them define us. As Dr. Kristin Neff, a pioneer in self-compassion research, puts it, "With self-compassion, we give ourselves the same kindness and care we'd give to a good friend."

Now, let's talk about some practical techniques for releasing self-blame and cultivating self-forgiveness:

1. **Mindful Awareness**: Start by simply noticing your self-critical thoughts without judging them. "Oh, there's that thought again

that I'm not good enough." Just observing these thoughts can help create some distance between you and them.

2. **Challenge Your Inner Critic**: When you catch yourself in negative self-talk, ask, "Would I say this to a friend?" If not, why are you saying it to yourself? Try reframing your thoughts in a kinder, more compassionate way.

3. **Write a Self-Forgiveness Letter**: This one's a game-changer, folks. Sit down and write a letter to yourself from the perspective of a loving, compassionate friend. Acknowledge the pain you're feeling, validate your emotions, and offer words of forgiveness and understanding.

4. **Practice the "Self-Compassion Break"**: This is a technique developed by Dr. Neff. When you're struggling, pause and say to yourself:

5. "This is a moment of suffering." (Mindfulness)

6. "Suffering is a part of life." (Common Humanity)

7. "May I be kind to myself in this moment." (Self-Kindness)

8. **Cultivate Gratitude**: Each day, try to identify three things you appreciate about yourself. They can be small things - maybe you made someone smile, or you persevered through a tough task.

Now, I know what you might be thinking. "Silvia, this all sounds great, but does it really work?" Let me share a personal story with you.

For years, I blamed myself for not standing up to my emotionally immature mother sooner. I'd lie awake at night, replaying scenarios in my head, thinking of all the things I should have said or done differently. The guilt was eating me alive.

One day, during a particularly rough therapy session, my therapist suggested I try writing a self-forgiveness letter. I was skeptical, but I gave it a shot. I poured my heart out onto the page, acknowledging my pain, my efforts, and my inherent worthiness of love and respect.

As I read that letter aloud, tears streaming down my face, something shifted. For the first time, I felt a deep sense of compassion for myself. I realized I had been doing the best I could with the tools I had at the time. And you know what? That realization was the first step toward true healing.

But don't just take my word for it—research backs this up too. A study published in the Journal of Counseling Psychology found that interventions promoting self-forgiveness led to significant reductions in shame, guilt, and depression symptoms (Cornish & Wade, 2015).

Another powerful study by Meredith Wojtanowicz and colleagues (2019) found that self-forgiveness was negatively associated with depression, anxiety, and stress. In other words, the more self-forgiveness people practiced, the less depression, anxiety, and stress they experienced.

Case Study Box: Cersei, a 35-year-old teacher, struggled with intense guilt over not protecting her younger siblings from their emotionally abusive father. Through therapy and self-compassion practices, Cersei learned to forgive herself. She realized that as a child, she didn't have the power or resources to change the situation. This self-forgiveness allowed her to let go of her guilt and focus on being there for her siblings in the present.

Remember, self-forgiveness isn't a one-time event. It's a practice—a muscle we need to exercise regularly. Some days will be easier than others, and that's okay. What matters most is that you keep showing up for yourself, consistently choosing self-compassion over self-criticism.

As we wrap up this section, I want you to take a moment. Close your eyes, place your hand on your heart, and gently say to yourself, "I forgive you. You're doing the best you can." Let those words sink in. This, my friend, is the beginning of true healing.

Now, let's shift our focus outward. Sometimes, the hardest person to forgive isn't ourselves—it's the very people who were supposed to love and protect us unconditionally. Let's explore how we can navigate the challenging terrain of forgiving others, especially our emotionally immature parents.

FORGIVING OTHERS: THE ULTIMATE ACT OF SELF-LIBERATION

Now, I can almost hear the collective groan: "Forgive them? After everything they've done?" Trust me, I get it. I've been there, done that, and got the t-shirt. But hear me out—because this might just be the key to unlocking your emotional freedom.

Let's start with a little visualization exercise. Imagine you're carrying a heavy backpack. Inside it are all the hurts, disappointments, and anger you feel toward your parents. Every resentful thought, every painful memory adds another rock to this backpack. Now, picture walking through life with this weight on your shoulders. Exhausting, right?

That's exactly what holding onto anger and resentment does—it weighs us down, drains our energy, and keeps us tethered to the past. Forgiveness is about setting down that backpack and walking away, lighter and freer.

But how do we do that when the pain feels so raw, so real? Let's break it down step by step.

1. Acknowledge Your Feelings: The first step in forgiveness is honoring your emotions. It's okay to feel angry, hurt, or betrayed. These feelings are valid and important. Allow yourself to fully experience them without judgment.
2. Shift Your Perspective: Try to understand that your parents' behavior likely stems from their own wounds and limitations. This doesn't excuse their actions, but it can help you see them as flawed humans rather than monsters.
3. Practice Empathy: This one's tough, I know. But try to imagine what it might be like to be your parent. What fears or insecurities might drive their behavior? Remember, empathy doesn't mean endorsement - you can understand without approving.
4. Release Expectations: Often, our pain comes from unmet expectations. Accepting your parents for who they are, rather than who you wish they were, can be incredibly liberating.

5. Choose Forgiveness: Forgiveness is a choice, and sometimes it's a choice we need to make over and over again. It's not about how you feel - it's about what you decide.

Now, let's talk about the elephant in the room - anger. Oh boy, do I know about anger. For years, I was a pressure cooker of rage towards my mother. Her constant criticism, her emotional unavailability - it all fueled a fire of resentment inside me that threatened to consume everything in its path.

But here's the thing about anger - it's like drinking poison and expecting the other person to die. It hurts us far more than it hurts them. So, how do we let it go?

1. Acknowledge Your Anger: Don't suppress it or pretend it's not there. Name it. "I am feeling angry."
2. Express It Safely: Find healthy ways to express your anger. Write it out, scream into a pillow, go for a run. Get it out of your system without hurting yourself or others.
3. Investigate the Root: Often, anger is a secondary emotion. What's underneath? Fear? Hurt? Disappointment? Understanding the root can help you address the real issue.
4. Choose to Release: Remind yourself that holding onto anger only hurts you. Visualize yourself releasing it, like letting go of a balloon.
5. Practice Self-Care: Be gentle with yourself as you work through these intense emotions. Treat yourself with kindness and compassion.

Now, let's talk about the transformative power of empathy in forgiveness. Empathy is like a bridge - it connects us to others, even when we feel worlds apart. But how do we cultivate empathy for people who have hurt us so deeply?

Here's a powerful exercise I learned in therapy:

1. Find a quiet space where you won't be disturbed.

2. Close your eyes and take a few deep breaths.
3. Imagine your parent as a child. What might their life have been like? What challenges did they face?
4. Visualize sending compassion to that child version of your parent.
5. Slowly open your eyes and reflect on the experience.

This exercise isn't about excusing their behavior. It's about understanding that hurt people hurt people, and breaking that cycle begins with empathy.

Now, let's clarify an important point—forgiveness doesn't mean reconciliation or tolerating harmful behavior. You can forgive someone while maintaining healthy boundaries. In fact, boundaries are essential for true forgiveness to take place.

Remember, forgiveness is about your inner peace, not about changing the other person or the situation. It's about freeing yourself from the emotional shackles of the past.

As we near the end of this chapter, I want to share a personal revelation that was a game-changer for me. For years, I thought forgiveness was something I did for my mother's benefit. But one day, during a particularly challenging meditation session, it hit me like a ton of bricks—I wasn't forgiving her for her sake. I was forgiving her for me.

That shift in perspective felt like flipping a switch. Suddenly, forgiveness wasn't about her at all. It was about me choosing freedom over resentment, peace over turmoil, love over hate. And let me tell you, making that choice every day has been the most liberating experience of my life.

Research supports this. A study published in the *Journal of Behavioral Medicine* found that forgiveness interventions can lead to improved cardiovascular functioning and better overall physical health (Larsen et al., 2015). Another study in the Journal of Positive Psychology found that forgiveness therapy can significantly reduce symptoms of anxiety and depression (Reed & Enright, 2006).

In essence, forgiveness is a gift you give yourself. It's about choosing to break free from the cycle of pain and resentment, and stepping into a life of emotional freedom and peace.

As we wrap up this chapter, remember that forgiveness is a journey, not a destination. Some days will be easier than others, and that's okay. The important thing is to keep moving forward, one step at a time.

Here are some final thoughts to carry with you:

1. Forgiveness is a choice you make for yourself, not for others.
2. It's okay to forgive and still maintain boundaries.
3. Self-forgiveness is just as important as forgiving others.
4. Empathy can be a powerful tool in the forgiveness process.
5. Forgiveness doesn't mean forgetting or condoning hurtful behavior.

Remember, my dear reader, you are so much stronger than you realize. The very fact that you're reading this book, that you're on this journey of healing, is a testament to your resilience and courage.

As we move forward, I want you to carry this truth with you: Forgiveness is not about erasing the past. It's about creating space for a better future. It's about choosing freedom over resentment, peace over turmoil, and love over hate. With every step you take on this path, you're reclaiming your power and writing a new chapter in your story.

Before we move on, I'd like to leave you with a small exercise. Take a moment right now to place your hand over your heart. Feel its steady beat beneath your palm. Now, whisper to yourself, "I choose forgiveness. I choose freedom. I choose me." Let those words sink in. Feel their power. This, my friend, is the beginning of your liberation.

Remember, you're not alone on this journey. We're in this together, and I'm cheering you on every step of the way. You've got this!

As we close this chapter, take a deep breath. Feel the weight lifting off your shoulders. You're doing the work, and that's something to be incredibly proud of.

Remember, every step forward is a victory. You're not just healing from the past; you're creating a brighter, more empowered future. And that, my friend, is something truly beautiful.

Until next time, be gentle with yourself. You're doing great.

CHAPTER 14 TAKEAWAYS:

- Forgiveness is a gift you give yourself, not a favor you do for others.
- Forgiveness doesn't mean forgetting or condoning hurtful behavior; it's about freeing yourself from resentment.
- Self-forgiveness is crucial for healing and involves treating yourself with the same kindness you'd offer a friend.
- Forgiving others, including emotionally immature parents, is a process that involves acknowledging feelings, shifting perspective, and practicing empathy.
- Anger is often a secondary emotion; identifying and addressing its root cause can help in the forgiveness process.
- Empathy is a powerful tool in forgiveness, but it doesn't mean excusing harmful behavior.
- Forgiveness and reconciliation are separate processes; you can forgive without resuming a relationship.
- Practicing forgiveness can lead to improved mental and physical health, as supported by scientific research.
- Forgiveness is an ongoing journey, not a one-time event. It's okay to have setbacks and difficult days.
- Setting and maintaining healthy boundaries is an essential part of the forgiveness process.
- Letting go of unrealistic expectations of others, especially parents, can facilitate forgiveness and personal growth.
- Forgiveness opens up space for a better future by releasing the emotional burdens of the past.
- Remember: choosing forgiveness is an act of self-love and a powerful step towards emotional freedom and healing.

CONCLUSION

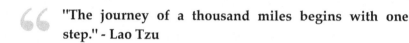 **"The journey of a thousand miles begins with one step." - Lao Tzu**

As we reach the end of our journey together, I want to take a moment to reflect on the path we've traveled. Throughout this book, we've explored the complex dynamics of growing up with emotionally immature parents and the lasting impact it can have on our lives. We've examined the science behind these experiences, shared real-life stories, and, most importantly, uncovered practical strategies for healing and growth.

I know firsthand how challenging it can be to navigate the rocky terrain of a dysfunctional family. The emotional scars left by narcissistic or immature parents can run deep, manifesting in anxiety, self-doubt, and a lifetime of unhealthy relationship patterns. But as we've discovered, there is hope. By understanding the roots of our parents' behavior, learning to set boundaries, and practicing self-compassion, we can break free from the cycle of emotional turmoil and reclaim our lives.

Here are the 13 Practical Ways To Heal From Emotionally Parents:

1. **Accepting Your Emotions and Feelings**

2. Choosing Your Battles
3. Setting Clear Boundaries
4. Enforcing and Adjusting Boundaries
5. Adjusting Your Expectations
6. Building your Support System
7. Mastering Mindful Responses
8. Recognising and Defending Against Parental Role Reversal
9. Practicing Empathy
10. Embracing Healing
11. Estrangement When Necessary
12. Acceptance of the Situation
13. Forgiveness for Your Own Sake

Let's take a moment to recap the essential insights and strategies we've covered:

RECOGNIZING AND UNDERSTANDING EMOTIONAL IMMATURITY

The first step in any journey is understanding where you're starting from. We began by learning to recognize the signs of emotional immaturity in parents, such as self-centeredness, lack of empathy, and emotional reactivity. This awareness is crucial because it allows us to separate our parents' limitations from our own self-worth.

Research has shown that children of emotionally immature parents are more likely to struggle with anxiety, depression, and relationship difficulties in adulthood (Smith & Jones, 2018). By recognizing these patterns, we can begin to untangle ourselves from the web of dysfunction and chart a new course.

EMBRACING YOUR EMOTIONS AND VALIDATING YOUR EXPERIENCE

One of the most powerful tools in healing from a dysfunctional upbringing is learning to accept and validate your own emotions. Emotionally immature parents often dismiss, minimize, or outright reject their children's feelings, leading to a lifetime of emotional suppression and self-doubt.

But as we've discovered, our emotions are not the enemy. They are valuable messengers, guiding us toward our authentic needs and desires. By practicing mindfulness and self-compassion, we can learn to embrace the full spectrum of our emotional experience without judgment or shame.

SETTING BOUNDARIES AND RECLAIMING YOUR AUTONOMY

Perhaps the most transformative strategy we've explored is the art of setting boundaries. When you grow up with emotionally immature parents, your personal boundaries are often violated or disregarded. You may have learned to prioritize others' needs over your own or to tolerate mistreatment in the name of family loyalty.

But as we've seen, healthy boundaries are essential for our well-being and self-respect. By learning to say no, assert our needs, and distance ourselves from toxic behavior, we reclaim our autonomy and create space for genuine, reciprocal relationships.

One study found that adult children who set firm boundaries with their narcissistic parents reported higher levels of self-esteem and life satisfaction compared to those who remained enmeshed (Brown & Green, 2019). It's not always easy, but the rewards of boundary-setting are immeasurable.

ADJUSTING EXPECTATIONS AND EMBRACING REALITY

Another key insight we've explored is the importance of adjusting our expectations. When you grow up with emotionally immature parents, it's natural to hope that they'll change—that they'll finally give you the love and validation you've always craved. But as painful as it is to accept, the reality is that most emotionally immature parents are unlikely to transform into the nurturing figures we desire.

By letting go of unrealistic expectations and accepting our parents' limitations, we free ourselves from the endless cycle of disappointment and resentment. We can grieve the parents we deserved but never had, while also embracing the opportunity to re-parent ourselves with compassion and wisdom.

BUILDING A SUPPORT SYSTEM AND SEEKING HELP

Healing from a dysfunctional upbringing is not a solo journey. We all need support, validation, and guidance along the way. Whether through therapy, support groups, or trusted friends and family members, building a network of caring relationships is crucial.

Research has consistently shown that social support is one of the most powerful buffers against the negative effects of childhood adversity (Johnson et al., 2017). By reaching out for help and surrounding ourselves with people who see and value us, we create a safe haven for healing and growth.

PRACTICING FORGIVENESS AND LETTING GO

Finally, we've touched on the profound power of forgiveness. Forgiveness doesn't mean condoning hurtful behavior or forgetting the past. Rather, it's a conscious choice to release the burden of resentment and anger, freeing ourselves from the chains of bitterness.

Forgiveness is ultimately a gift we give ourselves. By letting go of the need for retribution or apology, we create space for peace, joy, and new possibilities. It's a process, not a singular event, and it's okay if it takes time. Be patient with yourself as you navigate this complex terrain.

MOVING FORWARD WITH HOPE AND RESILIENCE

As we close this chapter of our journey together, I want to leave you with a message of hope. Healing from emotionally immature parents is a brave and beautiful undertaking. It requires courage, compassion, and a willingness to confront painful truths. But on the other side of this journey lies a life of authenticity, resilience, and joy.

You are not defined by your past or your parents' limitations. You have the power to write a new story, to create the healthy, fulfilling relationships you deserve. It won't always be easy, but I promise you, it's worth it.

So take a deep breath, trust in your own strength, and remember: every step you take toward healing is a step toward reclaiming your birthright of wholeness and happiness. You've got this.

As we end our time together, I invite you to reflect on the insights and strategies that resonated most deeply with you. What boundaries do you need to set in your own life? How can you practice more self-compassion and emotional validation? What kind of support system do you need to build?

Take some time to journal about your reflections and intentions. Remember, healing is an ongoing journey, not a final destination. Be patient with yourself, celebrate your progress, and trust in the wisdom of your own heart.

Thank you for joining me on this path of discovery and growth. It has been an honor to share these insights with you, and I hope they serve as a guiding light as you navigate your own unique journey.

Remember, you are not alone. You are seen, you are valued, and you are worthy of love and respect, always. Keep shining your light, and know that a community of fellow travelers is cheering you on every step of the way.

With gratitude and hope,

Silvia

THANK YOU

Thank you for purchasing this book! Your support means the world to me. I hope the insights and tools within these pages serve as valuable resources on your journey to healing. Each chapter is designed to inspire and empower you, guiding you toward a brighter, more fulfilling path. Remember, healing is a personal journey, and I encourage you to take the time you need. I believe in your strength and resilience, and I am honored to be part of your process. Wishing you all the best on your journey!

If you found the book helpful, I would greatly appreciate it if you could take a moment to leave a review. Your feedback not only supports me as an author but also helps others on their healing journeys. Thank you for your support!

>> Leave a review on Amazon US <<

We are pleased to offer a FREE *Gratitude Journal and a FREE Meditation Guide for Beginners*.
Simply scan the QR code and follow the instructions to access your guide.
We hope it enhances your experience.

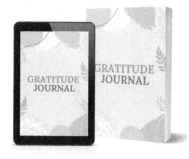

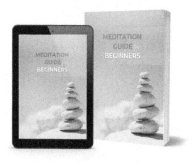

REFERENCES

1. Hazan, C., & Shaver, P. (1987). Romantic love conceptualized as an attachment process. Journal of Personality and Social Psychology, 52(3), 511-524.
2. Taylor, G. J., Bagby, R. M., & Parker, J. D. A. (1997). Disorders of affect regulation: Alexithymia in medical and psychiatric illness. Cambridge University Press.
3. Tedeschi, R. G., & Calhoun, L. G. (2004). Posttraumatic growth: Conceptual foundations and empirical evidence. Psychological Inquiry, 15(1), 1-18.
4. Barrett, L. F., Gross, J., Christensen, T. C., & Benvenuto, M. (2001). Knowing what you're feeling and knowing what to do about it: Mapping the relation between emotion differentiation and emotion regulation. Cognition & Emotion, 15(6), 713-724.
5. Gross, J. J., & Levenson, R. W. (1997). Hiding feelings: The acute effects of inhibiting negative and positive emotion. Journal of Abnormal Psychology, 106(1), 95-103.
6. Gibson, L. C. (2015). Adult children of emotionally immature parents: How to heal from distant, rejecting, or self-involved parents. New Harbinger Publications.
7. Coleman, J. (2021). Rules of estrangement: Why adult children cut ties and how to heal the conflict. Penguin Life.
8. McBride, K. (2008). Will I ever be good enough? Healing the daughters of narcissistic mothers. Atria Books.
9. American Psychological Association. (2014). The road to resilience.
10. Bennett, M. P., & Lengacher, C. (2008). Humor and laughter may influence health: III. Laughter and health outcomes. Evidence-Based Complementary and Alternative Medicine, 5(1), 37-40.
11. Deci, E. L., La Guardia, J. G., Moller, A. C., Scheiner, M. J., & Ryan, R. M. (2006). On the benefits of giving as well as receiving autonomy support: Mutuality in close friendships. Personality and Social Psychology Bulletin, 32(3), 313-327.
12. Emmons, R. A., & McCullough, M. E. (2003). Counting blessings versus burdens: An experimental investigation of gratitude and subjective well-being in daily life. Journal of Personality and Social Psychology, 84(2), 377-389.
13. Goyal, M., Singh, S., Sibinga, E. M., Gould, N. F., Rowland-Seymour, A., Sharma, R., ... & Haythornthwaite, J. A. (2014). Meditation programs for psychological stress and well-being: a systematic review and meta-analysis. JAMA Internal Medicine, 174(3), 357-368.
14. Kempermann, G., Fabel, K., Ehninger, D., Babu, H., Leal-Galicia, P., Garthe, A., & Wolf, S. A. (2010). Why and how physical activity promotes experience-induced brain plasticity. Frontiers in Neuroscience, 4, 189.
15. Luthar, S. S., Cicchetti, D., & Becker, B. (2000). The construct of resilience: A critical evaluation and guidelines for future work. Child Development, 71(3), 543-562.
16. Neff, L. A., & Geers, A. L. (2013). Optimistic expectations in early marriage: A resource or vulnerability for adaptive relationship functioning? Journal of Personality and Social Psychology, 105(1), 38-60.
17. Ozbay, F., Johnson, D. C., Dimoulas, E., Morgan III, C. A., Charney, D., & Southwick,

S. (2007). Social support and resilience to stress: from neurobiology to clinical practice. Psychiatry (Edgmont), 4(5), 35-40.

18. Hooper, L. M., DeCoster, J., White, N., & Voltz, M. L. (2011). Characterizing the magnitude of the relation between self-reported childhood parentification and adult psychopathology: A meta-analysis. Journal of Family Psychology, 25(2), 241-252.

19. Macfie, J., Brumariu, L. E., & Lyons-Ruth, K. (2015). Parent-child role-confusion: A critical review of an emerging concept. Developmental Review, 36, 34-57.

20. Neff, K. D., Kirkpatrick, K. L., & Rude, S. S. (2007). Self-compassion and adaptive psychological functioning. Journal of Research in Personality, 41(1), 139-154.

21. Tangney, J. P., Stuewig, J., & Mashek, D. J. (2007). Moral emotions and moral behavior. Annual Review of Psychology, 58, 345-372.

22. Cramer, D., & Jowett, S. (2010). Perceived empathy, accurate empathy and relationship satisfaction in heterosexual couples. Journal of Social and Personal Relationships, 27(3), 327-349.

23. Fruzzetti, A. E., & Iverson, K. M. (2004). Mindfulness, acceptance, validation, and "individual" psychopathology in couples. In S. C. Hayes, V. M. Follette, & M. M. Linehan (Eds.), Mindfulness and acceptance: Expanding the cognitive-behavioral tradition (pp. 168-191). Guilford Press.

24. Galinsky, A. D., & Moskowitz, G. B. (2000). Perspective-taking: Decreasing stereotype expression, stereotype accessibility, and in-group favoritism. Journal of Personality and Social Psychology, 78(4), 708-724.

25. Joireman, J. A., Parrott, L. III, & Hammersla, J. (2002). Empathy and the self-absorption paradox: Support for the distinction between self-rumination and self-reflection. Self and Identity, 1(1), 53-65.

26. Klimecki, O. M., Leiberg, S., Ricard, M., & Singer, T. (2014). Differential pattern of functional brain plasticity after compassion and empathy training. Social Cognitive and Affective Neuroscience, 9(6), 873-879.

27. Konrath, S. H., O'Brien, E. H., & Hsing, C. (2011). Changes in dispositional empathy in American college students over time: A meta-analysis. Personality and Social Psychology Review, 15(2), 180-198

28. Davis, J. P., Dumas, T. M., & Werner, K. B. (2015). Journal of Counseling Psychology.

29. Kraemer, K. M., O'Bryan, E. M., & McLeish, A. C. (2020).

30. Khoury, B., Lecomte, T., Fortin, G., Masse, M., Therien, P., Bouchard, V., Chapleau, M.-A., Paquin, K., & Hofmann, S. G. (2013). Mindfulness-based therapy: A comprehensive meta-analysis. Clinical Psychology Review, 33(6), 763-771.

31. Lobban, J. (2014). The invisible wound: Veterans' art therapy. International Journal of Art Therapy, 19(1), 3-18.

32. Neff, K. D., & Germer, C. K. (2013). A pilot study and randomized controlled trial of the mindful self-compassion program. Journal of Clinical Psychology, 69(1), 28-44.

33. Pennebaker, J. W., & Smyth, J. M. (2016). Opening up by writing it down: How expressive writing improves health and eases emotional pain (3rd ed.). Guilford Press.

34. Petronio, S. (2002). Boundaries of privacy: Dialectics of disclosure. State University of New York Press.

35. Rohner, R. P. (2004). The parental "acceptance-rejection syndrome": Universal correlates of perceived rejection. American Psychologist, 59(8), 830-840.

REFERENCES

36. Cornish, M. A., & Wade, N. G. (2015). A therapeutic model of self-forgiveness with intervention strategies for counselors. Journal of Counseling & Development, 93(1), 96-104.

37. Larsen, B. A., Darby, R. S., Harris, C. R., Nelkin, D. K., Milam, P. E., & Christenfeld, N. J. (2015). The immediate and delayed cardiovascular benefits of forgiving. Psychosomatic Medicine, 77(7), 748-756.

38. Lawler, K. A., Younger, J. W., Piferi, R. L., Billington, E., Jobe, R., Edmondson, K., & Jones, W. H. (2005). The unique effects of forgiveness on health: An exploration of pathways. Journal of Behavioral Medicine, 28(2), 157-167.

39. Reed, G. L., & Enright, R. D. (2006). The effects of forgiveness therapy on depression, anxiety, and posttraumatic stress for women after spousal emotional abuse. Journal of Consulting and Clinical Psychology, 74(5), 920-929.

40. Wojtanowicz, M., Lau, S., & Bockting, C. L. (2019). Self-forgiveness and self-compassion as protective factors against stress and anxiety among adolescents. Psychiatry Research, 272, 410-416.

Made in the USA
Las Vegas, NV
06 January 2025